2-31-93

Respiratory Anatomy and Physiology

Respiratory Anatomy and Physiology

David E. Martin, Ph.D.
Department of Cardiopulmonary
    Care Sciences
Georgia State University
Atlanta, Georgia

John W. Youtsey, Ph.D.
Series Editor

Faculty Lecture Series in Respiratory Care

THE C. V. MOSBY COMPANY
ST. LOUIS   TORONTO   WASHINGTON, D.C.

Executive Editor: David T. Culverwell
Production Coordinator: Lisa G. Cunninghis
Manuscript/Production Editor: A. Tony Meléndez
Art: Joe Vitek

Library of Congress Cataloging-in-Publication Data
Martin, David E., 1939–
    Respiratory anatomy and physiology.
    Includes bibliographies and index.
    1. Respiratory organs. 2. Respiratory organs—Anatomy. I. Title. [DNLM: 1. Respiratory System—anatomy & histology. 2. Respiratory System—physiology. WF 101 M379r]
QP121.M365   1987   612'.2   87-15299
ISBN 0-8016-3175-0

Printed in the United States of America

VH/VH   9 8 7 6 5 4 3 2 1   01/B/015

TABLE OF CONTENTS

FOREWORD

Respiratory Anatomy and Physiology represents the third book in the Faculty Lecture Series in Respiratory Care. Like the first two in the series, **Assessment of the Pulmonary Patient** and **Mechanical Ventilation: Physiological and Clinical Applications,** this text will serve as a valuable educational resource.

Anatomy and physiology of the respiratory system is the knowledge base upon which our clinical therapy is founded. Our understanding of respiratory diseases and disorders, therapeutic modalities, and patient evaluation would not be possible without a strong background in anatomy and physiology. The respiratory care practitioner, as well as the nurse and other health care practitioners, must be able to effectively integrate the theory knowledge with the clinical picture in order to appropriately manage the patient in today's complex health care technology.

Often times, traditional respiratory anatomy and physiology texts do not meet the needs of the health care practitioner. They are often written from the classical or traditional physiologist's perspective. Such is not the case with this text.

In *Respiratory Anatomy and Physiology,* Dr. David Martin has provided a unique and highly readable approach. The text is theoretically sound and written in such a manner that Dr. Martin's mastery over the subject matter and understanding of the medical arena are obvious. This text has been an evolutionary process based on over fifteen years of teaching experience with students in respiratory therapy, nursing, and medicine.

John W. Youtsey
Georgia State University
Atlanta, Georgia

PREFACE

This book follows the format of a lecture series delivered annually to students pursuing a Bachelor of Science degree with a specialty in respiratory therapy at Georgia State University. Experience indicates that this book may also have considerable value to other allied health science professionals as well, particularly nurses and cardiopulmonary technologists. The format has also proved useful for medical students desiring an easily readable overview of the anatomy and physiology of the pulmonary system.

It is presumed that students reading this book will have had some good basic college courses in chemistry, physics, and biology. All are essential to proceeding forward with an understanding of how the pulmonary system operates. Anatomic concepts are presented initially, to provide a structural framework on which to explain physiology, the science of function in living systems. No references to the vast literature of these subject matter areas are provided in the text, because this is not intended as an encyclopedic documentation. At the end of each chapter, however, a list of selected references identify some of the classic original papers, some newer review articles, and useful books on the subjects discussed. Readers can then delve more deeply into areas of special interest as desired.

The various organ systems of the body interact in myriad and marvelous ways. The pulmonary system interactions with several systems, notably blood, blood vessels, and the heart, are of enormous importance. Better understanding of, and appreciation for, pulmonary system function can often be enhanced by brief diversions into the workings of these other organ systems, and this occurs freely in the text. To appreciate the entire picture of lung function, one cannot any longer be pedantically narrow and restricted in focus. To do so is to become too compartmentalized, and unable to communicate with those whose related interests are germane and crucial to that whole picture. At an early level, students in the health care professions must be stimulated to look beyond a narrow focus, for it will better allow them to interact beneficially with their colleagues in the health care system. Aspects of histology, pathology, and biochemistry are thus also discussed wherever they can be effective in enhancing an appreciation for pulmonary structure and function.

David E. Martin, Ph D
Professor
Department of
Cardiopulmonary Care Sciences
Georgia State University
Atlanta, Georgia

ACKNOWLEDGMENTS

A debt of appreciation goes first to the many students who, over the years, have had to work with various drafts of these chapters as teaching materials for their course in respiratory anatomy and physiology. Their encouragement and suggestions for improvement aided greatly in the timely completion of this endeavor. The majority of the manuscript was typed initially by Ms. Leigh Walling in my Department. Specific sections of the manuscript were scrutinized by William A. Guest, RRT, MD, now practicing in Tifton, Georgia. Scanning electron micrographs of primate tissues were prepared by Mr. Bill McManus while at the Yerkes Primate Research Center of Emory University. The remainder of the illustrations and graphs have been either created by the excellent medical illustration staff of The C. V. Mosby Company or reprinted from their original sources with permission, thereby giving recognition to the excellence with which other authors have tackled the never-ceasing dilemma of how best to picture an important concept. The author welcomes any suggestions that may focus further on improvements to make this text more useful and enjoyable as a tool for learning.

The Respiratory System: General Principles

Chapter One

Chapter One Outline

The main function of respiration is to provide oxygen (O_2) to the cells of the body and to remove excess carbon dioxide (CO_2) from them. Because of the size and complexity of organ systems in multicellular animals, a sophisticated gas exchange system is essential. The mechanisms explaining how the lungs and associated structures accomplish this in humans is the subject of human respiratory physiology.

It is the purpose of this book to consider the anatomy and physiology of the respiratory system. The study of anatomy emphasizes structure, while that of physiology emphasizes function. Structure and function work hand in hand. A structurally superior respiratory system would imply that the individual possessing it might have increased functional abilities. Similarly, with disease processes, defects in organ structure may adversely affect the function of the organs, whereas defects in function can affect organ system structure.

GENERAL CONCEPTS OF PHYSIOLOGICAL REGULATION

To more fully appreciate and understand the function of the respiratory system, it is useful at the outset to create a familiarity with the general concepts by which living systems maintain their functional integrity. Two interrelated concepts are those of *simplicity* and *specificity*. At first glance, the several thousand different macromolecules comprising living tissues may appear exceedingly complex. However, the general organization of living systems has some simple and specific features. Every cell type (except a very few highly specialized such as the red blood cell) has a nucleus surrounded by cytoplasm. Most cells possess the potential for continuing existence by division or replication. Organic chemical reactions involving these macromolecules proceed similarly in all cells.

All the macromolecules are constructed from the same building blocks: amino acids, sugars and fatty acids. The macromolecules all have specific functions, thus providing specificity to the cells. In an informative book published in 1972 entitled *Biological Order*, Andre Lwoff, a French physiologist wrote: "the machine is built for doing precisely what it does. We may admire it, but we should not lose our heads. If the living system did not perform its task, it would not exist. We have simply to learn how it performs its task."

A third concept is one of the very cornerstones of physiological structure—the idea of *constancy* within the environment bathing cells of multi-cellular organisms. Claude Bernard, often referred to as the father of the discipline of physiology, in 1878 described the idea of constancy as follows:

"animals have really two environments: a milieu exterieur in which the organism is situated, and a milieu interieur, in which the tissue elements live. The living organism does not really exist in the milieu exterieur (the atmosphere if it breathes, salt or fresh water if that is its element), but in the liquid milieu interieur formed by the circulating organic liquid which surrounds and bathes all the tissue elements. This is the lymph or plasma, the liquid part of the blood which, in the higher animals is diffused through the tissues and forms the ensemble of the intercellular liquids and is the basis of all local nutrition and the common factor of all elementary exchanges. The stability of the milieu interieur is the primary condition for freedom and independence of existence."

Nearly 50 years after Bernard's concept of keeping the internal environment constant, Harvard University physiology professor Walter B. Cannon emphasized that this cellular maintenance occurs by constant tearing down and building up of the various macromolecules within living systems. Thus, an overall steady state is achieved through constant change. In a small book entitled *The Wisdom of the Body,* Cannon wrote that

"the coordinated physiological processes which maintain most of the steady states in the organism are so complex and so peculiar to living beings . . . that I have suggested a special designation for these states, *homeostasis.* The word does not imply something set and immobile, a stagnation. It means a condition—a condition which may vary, but which is relatively constant."

A good working definition for homeostasis is those dynamic, self-regulating processes that maintain an essentially constant internal environment. As an example, loss of water initiates thirst; this results in the ingestion of fluid which compensates for the body water lost. The control of such processes is largely through negative feedback, a mechanism whereby a stimulus initiating the physiological compensatory process is removed after the previous equilibrium is regained.

A fifth guiding concept involves that of *activity,* and its chief exponent was the British physiologist Joseph Barcroft. *The condition of rest,* he wrote in *Features in the Architecture of Physiological Function,* "is the essence of the machine." Humans, just as with other species, have not evolved yet into motionless, idling creatures. Instead, they have enormous performance potential that can and must constantly be developed and challenged. By frequent vigorous physical activity, ongoing basal activities can be carried out with greater relative ease. Barcroft's favorite example was a giant train locomotive standing in a railroad station, with its engine idling, and one could only imagine its true capabilities when pulling dozens of loaded freight cars at high speed. The enormous capabilities of the respiratory system, at rest and during exercise, are analogous to those of the locomotive, and will be described in this text.

Finally, the principles of *adaptation* and *symmorphosis* are important. When organ systems are challenged, homeostatic mechanisms allow not only an immediate response to the altered environmental situation, but also, in many instances, a long-term adaptation of positive benefit. People who ascend to high altitude will, after several days, increase their O_2–carrying abilities as an adaption to the continuing low O_2 levels in the inspired air. They do this by increasing their circulating numbers of red blood cells, and thus their blood hemoglobin. Long distance runners increase the number and size of mitochondria in their skeletal muscles as an adaptation to their arduous training. This improves their fuel utilization and O_2–extraction capabilities. The concept of symmorphosis explains the extent of the adaptation: it will not be in excess of needs, rather only sufficient to meet the imposed challenge.

EVOLUTION OF THE AIR-BREATHING MECHANISM

In studying respiration we are studying probably the single most significant element of change in the evolutionary history of the vertebrates—the adoption of an air breathing system which allowed departure from a water environment in favor of a terrestrial one. This migration from the sea to land began to occur about 350 million years ago. Climatic conditions produced large masses of warm, shallow, and turbid fresh water which covered a great portion of the earth. In warm and stagnant water, gases are not dissolved nearly as readily as when the water temperature is lower and the gases are bubbled through it. Thus these water masses were O_2–deficient. The contemporary fishes of the time adapted by evolving into air breathers while they were still aquatic. This occurred long before they were able to adapt permanently as terrestrial species (Figure 1-1).

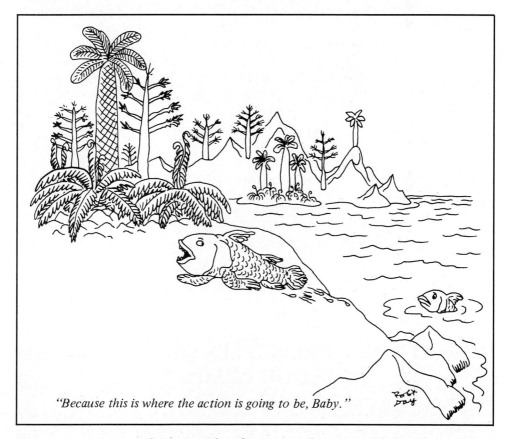

"Because this is where the action is going to be, Baby."

Figure 1-1.   Cartoon depiction of evolutionary adaptation of fishes from a water-breathing to an air-breathing existence. Reprinted with permission from The New Yorker Vol. 42 (13): p. 53, 21 May 1966.

In the context of evolution, the important physiologic point here is that O_2 absorption by these organisms became independent of water much earlier than did CO_2 elimination. The later evolution of CO_2 riddance is credited to at least a 20–fold greater solubility of CO_2 than O_2 in water, which favors CO_2 escape at any air-water (alveolar lining layer) surface bordering the ambient environment. There is a great benefit in such a movement of organisms from a water to an air environment, particularly regarding O_2 transport. Air can hold about 30 times more O_2 molecules per unit of volume than water. Oxygen has a coefficient of diffusion about 10,000 times greater in air than in water. Taken together, these physical facts suggest that O_2 can move into O_2–utilizing tissues thousands of times faster if they are in air than in water. Water is 60 times more viscous than air and its smaller O_2–carrying capacity forces water dwellers to constantly keep water moving past their gas exchange apparatus (such as gills in a fish) to prevent buildup of an O_2–poor fluid layer. Although no system is perfect, and the air breathers must constantly contend with dehydration as a result of water loss from their exposed moist gas exchange organs, still the air breathing mechanism is ultimately more efficient.

It is equally significant that blood flow in the various evolving species is lowest in those species having the highest hemoglobin concentration. We will learn that hemoglobin is a remarkable O_2–carrying molecule in terms of quantitative transport ability. This suggests that blood flow is adjusted in part to match the O_2–carrying status of the blood.

Ventilation and circulation in living organisms both require metabolic energy. With increasing body size, accommodating these physiologic processes presents a formidable challenge. The transition to active terrestrial life was thus associated with an increase in O_2–carrying capacity (via hemoglobin), beyond that which could be physically dissolved in plasma, and an increased buffering ability of the blood to counter metabolic acidosis. (This is acidosis in which excess acid is added to the body fluids or bicarbonate is lost from them.) These combined adaptations have provided an efficiency of gas transport which surpasses that which could be provided by increased ventilation and perfusion alone. The task of the remaining chapters is to explain the details of these physiologic mechanisms.

OPERATIONAL PRINCIPLES OF THE AIR AND BLOOD PUMPS

The pumps which circulate air and blood differ quite markedly. The right ventricle of the heart pushes blood unidirectionally into the lungs. Backflow is prevented by valves. The air pump differs by not having valves—it moves air back and forth through the same set of conducting tubes. No gas exchange with the blood occurs from these conducting tubes, and thus their volume is often referred to collectively as anatomical dead space. This dead space is both good and bad. Thus, with so much surface area not usable for diffusion, more ventilation is needed. This means more ventilatory work. However, the two-way nature of the gas-conducting system permits more space in the lungs for diffusion of gases by eliminating the need for a separate set of collecting tubes for expired gases.

Another important difference between the two pumps lies in their generation of pressure. The blood pump (the heart) is a positive pressure pump. Positive pressure is compressed air or gas that is delivered to the respiratory passages at greater than ambient pressure. Tension generated in cardiac muscle pushes blood out of its chambers, and relaxation allows blood to enter. The thoracic pump, by contrast, is a negative pressure pump—flow is from outside to inside. By enlarging its capacity, the pressure in alveoli is lowered to less than atmospheric pressure. Fresh air then flows in the direction of outside the lungs to inside the lungs (i.e., down its pressure gradient). Exhalation becomes a passive process, resulting from recoil of the lungs.

Similarities also exist between the pumps. Both pumps are variable performance devices. Both are regulated with exquisite precision to meet body needs with the least energy cost. The discipline of respiratory physiology attempts to demonstrate: 1) how this normal precision is managed, 2) how this precision allows one to adapt to variations in environmental gas concentrations and humidity, and 3) how abnormalities in this precision result in pathologic consequences.

In essence the maintenance of adequate cardiopulmonary function requires:

1. Optimum provision of the lungs with air to permit adequate gas exchange with blood, i.e., O_2 entry into the blood and CO_2 riddance from it—*ventilation*.
2. Optimum diffusion of these gases between lung and blood—a functional *alveolocapillary membrane*.
3. Optimum capillary circulation to ensure that the alveoli can exchange gases with the blood—*perfusion*.
4. Optimum ability to get the gases to and from the body tissues via the bloodstream—*transport*.

DYNAMICS OF THE RESPIRATORY SYSTEM

A one-celled organism floating in water requires no elaborate apparatus to extract O_2 from its surroundings. Its needs are satisfied by the process of diffusion—a random movement of molecules that results in a net flow of O_2 from the region of abundance around it to regions of scarcity within its cytoplasm. Over very short distances, such as through a cell, O_2 diffusion is rapid. Over larger distances, O_2 diffusion is a much slower process. The larger organisms become, the greater is their mass in relation to their surface area. Even under optimal conditions, assuming a completely spherical organism, the mass increases directly as the cube of its radius (r^3), whereas the surface area increases as the square of its radius (r^2). Diffusion cannot meet the needs of a multicellular organism in which the distance between the source of O_2 and the most remote cell is greater than about a millimeter. Some kind of circulating system is essential, and the vast array of more primitive organisms such as sponges, sea anemones, and worms achieve this in diverse ways.

Large animals, particularly the more highly evolved mammals living on land, make use of two systems: 1) an air pump consisting of the thoracic cage and lungs, and 2) a fluid pump system consisting of the heart and vascular system. The lungs with their airways have more contact area with the external environment than any other organ of the body. The air pump takes in air and exposes it to the circulating blood, which is specialized (largely by the presence of hemoglobin molecules) for storing large quantities of gases. In this way gas transport goes efficiently to and from all cells of the various metabolizing tissues. The key to the functioning of this system is a set of membranes allowing very close apposition of components of the two systems for the purpose of gaseous exchange. Thus in the lung the primary air-carrying tubes branch into thousands of smaller tubes finally ending as alveoli. With walls only one cell layer thick, many alveoli are almost directly apposed to capillary walls.

These capillary walls are also only one cell layer thick. The capillary is the one place in the circulatory system where diffusion across the walls of the vessel can occur. The blood pump essentially drives the entire output of the right heart through these pulmonary capillaries. The phrase "mixed venous blood" is often used to describe the blood coming from the right heart to the lungs. It is a mixture. Blood returning from each of the many systemic vessel beds of the body will have varying amounts of O_2 remaining and CO_2 added, depending on the metabolic activity in each of these beds. When this blood enters the right heart from the superior or inferior vena cava, it mixes together. This "mixed venous blood" then travels to the lung via the pulmonary artery. When it courses through the pulmonary capillaries, O_2 will be added and CO_2 removed. This richly oxygenated blood will then return to the left heart via the pulmonary vein (Figure 1-2).

Even though this principle of cardiopulmonary interaction is easily understood, one must never forget the incredible complexity of these two systems. Let us assume a normal respiratory rate of about 12 breaths per minute. With each breath about a half a liter of air is inspired. At the end of a day an individual would have taken 12 breaths/min × 60 minutes/hr × 24 hr/day = 17,280 breaths and will have inspired 500 milliliters/breath × 17,280 breaths/day = 8,640 liters of air. All of this air swirls through a maze of breathing ducts, from mouth and nose into the depths of the lungs. About 70% eventually ventilates the 300 million air sacs called alveoli. These alveoli are part of a gas exchange apparatus along with pulmonary capillaries. Approximately 21% of the inspired air is

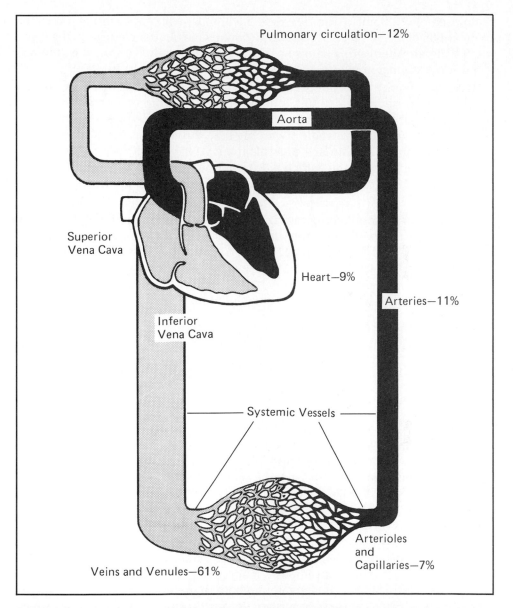

Pulmonary circulation—12%

Aorta

Superior
Vena Cava

Heart—9%

Arteries—11%

Inferior
Vena Cava

Systemic Vessels

Arterioles
and
Capillaries—7%

Veins and Venules—61%

Figure 1-2. Diagram to show the location of highly oxygenated (systemic arterial and pulmonary venous) blood as compared with the lesser oxygenated (systemic venous and pulmonary arterial) blood in the cardiovascular system. Rapid oxygenation of blood occurs as it courses through the pulmonary capillaries. Blood in the right heart and pulmonary artery is often termed 'mixed venous' blood, since it is a mixture of blood, with varying amounts of oxygen removed, returning from various tissue beds via the superior and inferior venae cavae.

composed of O_2. Some of the O_2 enters the bloodstream, for eventual use in the metabolism of foods. The CO_2 resulting from this metabolism returns to the lungs via the blood. After gas exchange has occurred, the inspired air must exit by the same route it entered before another volume can be brought in.

At rest we require a transfer of 200 ml to 250 ml of O_2 into the body per minute. Maximal exercise may raise this to more than 5,000 ml/min. At rest, we must deliver fresh air through the lungs in sufficient quantity to almost simultaneously ventilate 300 million alveoli of varying size through a million tubes. These alveoli will provide a surface area of about 160 m². Diffusion through the alveolocapillary membrane, which is 1.0 μm thick, will allow the addition of O_2 and removal of sufficient quantities of CO_2 to ensure the metabolic well-being of the organism.

The engineering problems of the circulatory system are equally impressive. As little as 4 liters of blood per minute at rest, or as much as 30 to 40 liters per minute during exercise, can be pumped by the heart in an adult. The capillary bed of the lungs has a surface area of about 158 m² with a wall thickness of not much more than 0.5 μm. The resistance to flow of blood through this bed is low. Normally, a driving pressure of less than 15 millimeters of mercury (mmHg) is adequate to produce flow.

STANDARDS FOR MEASUREMENT: THE SI SYSTEM

Consistency in the format by which measured respiratory data are reported is crucial for accurate communication of such data. Since several systems of units for expressing values in respiratory physiology are used, this has not been achieved worldwide. For at least three reasons, reluctance to change in such matters is sizable. There is the economic burden imposed upon the particular generation that decides to change from one system of notation to another. Another problem involves the restructuring of automated thinking that develops as one grows into any particular system gradually. For example, changing from feet and inches to meters and centimeters requires conscious effort. Finally, some measurements are more conveniently made using one system, some using another, thus creating the desire to maintain both in preference to complete consistency. A brief discussion of the systems of units relevant to respiratory physiology is appropriate. These units will be used throughout this text.

Three fundamental units of measurement were established during the time period of the French Revolution. *Length* in centimeters, *mass* in grams, and *time* in seconds were adopted by most scientific and industrialized nations. Notable exceptions to the use of this so-called CGS (centimeter-gram-second) system included the English-speaking nations, which preferred the inch for length and the pound for mass.

Beginning in 1960 an International System of units was promulgated worldwide. At this time, the *meter* and the *kilogram* were substituted, respectively, for the centimeter and gram. This system is referred to as the MKS (meter-kilogram-second) system. Physicists and chemists simultaneously recommended the use of the mole for *quantity* of a substance. The term "SI Units" refers to the French "Le Système International d'Unités." The entry of Great Britain into the European Economic Community during the 1970s resulted in the British adoption of SI units, leaving the United States of America as the only major nonconforming nation. During the decade of the 1980s a trend toward conversion to the SI units emerged within the United States. This change is becoming even more apparent in many areas of business and technology.

From these SI base units, other units can be derived. They have names which have been assigned to honor the great men whose research pioneered the areas of science most relevant to the unit's use. Several of these will be utilized in this text, and they are summarized in Table 1-1. For example, when we explore the problem of surface tension in alveoli we will encounter the unit of force—the *Newton* (N)—which is one kilogram-meter per second per second (1 kg–m/s^2). Surface tension is measured in newtons/m. The newton replaces the *dyne*, which is one gram centimeter per second per second (1 gm–cm/s^2). Thus 1 N = 10^5 dynes and 1 dyne = 0.00001 N or, 1 millinewton per meter (1 mN/m) = one dyne/centimeter (1 dyne/cm). Additional units, such as the milliliter, liter, minute and standard atmosphere are not included as SI units, but have practical value and hence are used when appropriate.

Discussion of metabolism involves heat production as part of free energy generated from catabolism of fuels. The appropriate unit here is the *joule* (J). One joule equals one newton-meter (1 J = 1 Nm). Thus one joule replaces the previously used *calorie* (cal) for heat and energy. One joule = 0.239 calories, and 1 cal = 4.18 J. One kilocalorie (kcal) = 4.18 kilojoules (kJ). This energy can be utilized for the performance of work. The time rate of performing work involves the concept of *power*, measured in *watts*. Thus, 1 watt = 1 joule/sec = 1Nm/sec.

The measurement of fluid and gas pressure is frustrating for many pulmonary physiologists when SI units are substituted for the more familiar unit of millimeters of mercury (mmHg.) While still a student in medical school, the now-famous physician, Jean Leonard Marie Poiseuille, pioneered investigations of arterial blood pressure on a standing mercury column based upon the concept of pressure defined as force per unit area. To this day, a simpler, more accurate system has not been devised for measuring blood pressure. For this reason the medical community has been reluctant to discontinue the unit of mmHg. Standardization in SI units should end the confusion of measuring cerebrospinal fluid pressure in mm H$_2$O and venous pressure in cm H$_2$O, which are also gravity-based systems.

The unit of *Torr* approximates one mmHg because it is 1/760 of a standard atmosphere. That unit's name honors the Italian physicist, Evangelista Torricelli. It is not an SI unit, however. Since pressure is defined as force per unit area, the proper SI description is newton per square meter (N/m^2). The assigned SI unit is the *pascal* (Pa), where 1 Pa = 1 N/m^2. This converts unevenly into mmHg such

Table 1-1. Summary of Some SI and Other Units.

Physical Quantity	SI Unit	Symbol	Definition of SI Unit	Other Common Unit	SI Conversion
Volume	Cubic meter	—	m^3		
Force	Newton	N	$1\ N = 1\ kg\ m/s^2$	dyne	$10^5\ dynes = 1\ N$
Pressure	Pascal	Pa	$1\ Pa = 1\ N/m^2$ $= 1\ kg/m\ s^2$	mmHg; cm H_2O	$1\ mmHg - 133.3\ Pa$ $= 0.133\ kPa$ $1\ kPa = 7.5\ mmHg$ $= 10.2\ cm\ H_2O$
Work, energy, heat	Joule	J	$1\ J = 1\ N\ m$ $= 1\ kg\ m^2/s^2$	calorie	$1\ J = 0.239\ cal;$ $1\ cal = 4.18\ J$
Power	Watt	W	$1\ W = 1\ N\ m/s$ $= 1\ J/s$		
Surface tension	Pascal meter	—	$1\ Pa\ m = 1\ N/m$ $= 1\ kg/s^2$	dyne/cm	$1\ dyne/cm$ $= 1\ mN/m$

$1\ cm\ H_2O = 0.736\ mmHg$
$1\ mmHg = 1.359\ cm\ H_2O$

that 1 mmHg $= 133.322$ Pa $= 0.133$ kilopascal (kPa). Or, 1 kPa $= 7.5$ mmHg $= 10.2$ cm H_2O. The often quoted normal healthy young adult blood pressure value of 120 mmHg systolic/80 mmHg diastolic pressure thus converts roughly to 16/11 kPa. Standard sea level barometric pressure of 760 mmHg is approximately 100 kPa (actually 101.3 kPa). Because of the present-day transition in systems of units routinely used, mmHg (also cm H_2O) and kPa will both be given in this book to provide familiarity with the two systems.

There is another unit for measuring pressure which is more frequently used by meteorologists, and that is the *millibar* (mbar). Since 1 mbar $= 100$ Pa (1 hecto-pascal or 1hPa), then 1 mmHg $= 1.33$ mbar.

Finally, some comment is appropriate concerning the use of the mole (M) for the quantity of a substance instead of the more familiar milliliter (ml) or liters (L) for gases. Using the principle developed by Amedeo Avogadro in the 19th century, one millimole (mM) of an ideal gas (such as O_2 or N_2) $= 22.39$ ml under standard conditions (STPD). Thus, 223.9 ml $= 10$mM. For non-ideal gases such as CO_2, 1mM $= 22.26$ ml.

Clinicians and clinical chemists often express quantities in terms of 100 ml blood. This is referred to either as volumes per cent (vol%) or deciliters (dl). Thus, arterial blood O_2 content is normally 20 ml/100 ml or 20 vol% or 20 ml/dl. Using SI notation, 20 ml O_2/100 ml blood becomes (20 ml/100 ml) $\times$ (0.045 mM/ml) $= 0.90$ mM/100 ml blood $= 9.0$mM/L). The situation regarding CO_2 is more complex. A large fraction of the blood CO_2 content is carried as bicarbonate (HCO_3^-), measured in mEq/L, where mM $=$ mEq/oxidation state (for HCO_3^-, mM $=$ mEq). Another fraction is CO_2 dissolved in the plasma and red blood cell water, typically measured in mM/L or ml/100 ml.

THE LANGUAGE OF RESPIRATORY PHYSIOLOGY

Since 1950, pulmonary physiologists have been quite consistent about using a precise set of terms that not only allows accurate communication but which also provides for easy transition from general discussion into mathematical expression. Symbols, used in precise format and sequence, allow conveyance of information simply and efficiently. These symbols must be learned early, with the reward being effective communication.

Primary symbols appear first, and are capital letters. They are as follows:

F $=$ fractional concentration of dry gas

P $=$ pressure of a gas (in blood or air)

C $=$ content of a gas in blood

Q $=$ volume of blood

S $=$ percent saturation of hemoglobin with O_2 or CO_2

D $=$ diffusing capacity

Secondary symbols appear as subscripts after the primary symbols. These are descriptive as to location or type of gas. They are as follows:

L = lung
I = inspired gas
E = expired gas
A = alveolar gas
D = deadspace gas
T = tidal gas
B = barometric
a = arterial blood
v = venous blood
c = capillary blood
s = shunted blood

Tertiary symbols are usually abbreviations for gases and again further describe the entity being symbolized. The most commonly discussed gases are the following:

O_2 = oxygen
CO_2 = carbon dioxide
CO   = carbon monoxide
N_2 = nitrogen
He   = helium

Two small symbols, a dot and a bar, may appear over the primary or secondary symbols. The dot signifies time and implies that the units of the particular symbol will have a time component. Thus, $\dot{V}O_2$ represents not just volume of O_2 in some quantity but rather volume of O_2 in a specific quantity per unit of time. Similarly, the bar represents an average or mean value. Thus $S\bar{v}O_2$ indicates the saturation of hemoglobin with O_2 in the mixed venous blood, that is, pooled blood from everywhere in the body, best obtained from the right ventricle.

Some examples of this symbolism are provided below to suggest the kinds of expressions that frequently appear both in this book and in the literature. Experience in using this terminology will remove its seeming complexity, and will greatly facilitate expression of ideas.

P_aCO_2 = partial pressure of carbon dioxide in blood
$\dot{V}_A/\dot{Q}_C$ = ratio of alveolar ventilation to pulmonary blood flow
SaO_2 = percent of saturation of hemoglobin with oxygen in arterial blood
V_T = tidal volume
P_B = barometric pressure
F_IN_2 = fraction of the inspired air that is nitrogen
$F_IO_2 \times \dot{V}_I$ = total inspired oxygen in ml/min

$F_EO_2 \times \dot{V}_E$ = total expired oxygen in ml/min

$\dot{V}O_2$ = oxygen consumption in ml/min = $(F_IO_2 \times \dot{V}_I) - (F_EO_2 \times \dot{V}_E)$

$C\bar{v}O_2$ = content of oxygen in mixed venous blood

D_LCO = diffusing capacity of the lung for carbon monoxide

RELEVANT READING

Barcroft, J. *Features in the Architecture of Physiological Function.* Cambridge Univ. Press, 1934.

Baron, D.N., Broughton, P.M.G., Cohen, M., Lansley, T.S., Lewis, S.M., and Shinton, N.K. The use of SI units in reporting results obtained in hospital laboratories. *Journal of Clinical Pathology,* **27:**590–597, 1974.

Bernard, C. In *Selected Readings in the History of Physiology,* (J.E. Fulton and L.G. Wilson, eds.), C.C. Thomas, Publ., Springfield, p. 326, 1966.

Cannon, W.B. *The Wisdom of the Body.* W.W. Norton & Co. Inc., New York, p. 24, 1963.

Cotes, J.E. SI units in respiratory medicine. *American Review of Respiratory Disease,* **112:**753–755, 1975.

Johansen, K. Cardiorespiratory adaptations in the transition from water breathing to air breathing. *Federation Proceedings* **29:**1118–1119, 1970.

Lwoff, A. *Biological Order.* M.I.T. Press, Cambridge, p. 13, 1962.

Padmore, G.R.A. and Nunn, J.F. SI units in relation to anaesthesia. *British Journal of Anaesthesia,* **46:**236–243, 1974.

Pappenheimer, J.R. Standardization of definitions and symbols in respiratory physiology. *Federation Proceedings,* **9:**602–605 1950.

Pierson, D.J. The evolution of breathing. 1. Introduction—why comparative physiology? *Respiratory Care* **27:**51–54, 1982.

Pierson, D.J. The evolution of breathing. 2. The nature of the problem. *Respiratory Care* **27:**160–163, 1982.

Pierson, D.J. The evolution of breathing. 3. Viable solutions: types of respiratory apparatus in animals. *Respiratory Care* **27:**267–270, 1982.

Pierson, D.J. The evolution of breathing. 6. Getting by with diffusion: animals with no breathing organs. *Respiratory Care* **27:**1063–1069, 1982.

Piiper, J., Dejours, P., Haab, P. and Rahre, M. Concepts and basic quantities in gas exchange physiology. *Respiration Physiology* **13:**292–304, 1971.

Rose, J.C. Pressures on the millimeter of mercury. *New England Journal of Medicine* **298:**1361–1364, 1978.

Vogel, S. Organisms that capture currents. *Scientific American* **239** (8): 128–139, 1978.

Young, D.S. Standardized reporting of laboratory data. *New England Journal of Medicine* **290:**368–373, 1974.

Gross Anatomy of the Respiratory System

Chapter Two

Chapter Two Outline

The respiratory system allows interchange of gases between the ambient environment and the bloodstream. This is sometimes termed *external respiration,* or more simply, breathing, to distinguish it between *internal respiration* (the actual exchange of gases between the blood and living cells) and *cellular respiration* (the oxidation of energy-producing fuels using one of the major inspired gases, O_2, with production of CO_2). A great variety of body tissues are involved in this external gas transfer: parts of the skeleton, muscles and nerves, and complex passageways that have other functions totally unrelated to ventilation, such as phonation, swallowing, and olfaction. A gross examination of these structures will provide an adequate basis for understanding their function in gas delivery to the blood. A more detailed understanding will lay a foundation for better appreciation of how pathological derangement in structure can adversely affect respiration.

THE NOSE AND PHARYNX

During breathing when the mouth is closed, air initially enters the respiratory tract via the two *external nares* or nostrils of the nose. *(Figure 2-1).* No one seems to understand clearly what determines whether we breathe through the nose or mouth, particularly when resistance to flow through the nose is greater than through the mouth. During exercise the oral route is utilized primarily. Neonates are obligatory nose breathers; perhaps their nasal resistance is less than that of adults in relation to their total airflow requirements. Although the shape of the nose itself—its breadth and length—varies considerably among ethnic groups, this has little influence on air movement through the two nostrils. The nares can be widened voluntarily by muscle action, but ordinarily this does not occur as a part of resting breathing. There are good reasons, however, for nasal breathing at rest being of greater functional value than oral breathing. First, the highly vascularized nasal passageways permit better humidification and heating or cooling of inspired air. Second, coarse hairs in the nasal vestibule, and cilia in the nasal cavities further along filter the inspired air. Third, the olfactory region helps determine whether the inspired air is of appropriate quality for the lungs. Noxious gases or particulate material can trigger a sniffing response. If the air is sufficiently polluted, a sneeze may result as the tract attempts to clean itself.

The nostrils come together 2 to 3 cm into the nose, forming two parallel *nasal cavities.* The 2 tubes are separated by a thin median cartilaginous *nasal septum,* and they extend another 4 to 5 cm to the pharynx. This is most easily seen in an X-ray of the head *(Figure 2-2).* The floor of this cavity is the palate; the roof is the delicate cribriform plate of the ethmoid bone, through which olfactory nerve fibers pass enroute to the brain. The lateral walls of the cavity are quite irregular, and are comprised not only of additional parts of the ethmoid bone (the superior and middle nasal conchae), but also a separate bone (the inferior nasal concha) articulating with the maxillary bone. Sometimes these conchae are referred to as turbinates, because of their scroll-shaped appearance when viewed from within

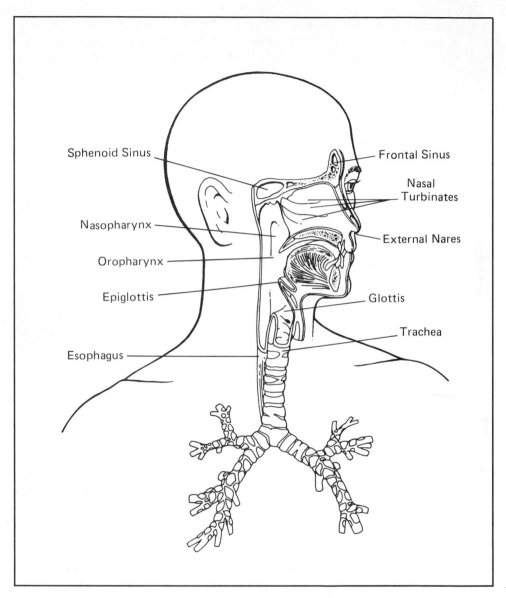

Sphenoid Sinus

Frontal Sinus

Nasal
Turbinates

Nasopharynx

External Nares

Oropharynx

Epiglottis

Glottis

Trachea

Esophagus

Figure 2-1   Sketch of upper thorax, neck, and head to illustrate general anatomical relationships of upper airway structures.

the nasal cavity (Figure 2-2). The cavity is very narrow, perhaps 1 mm to 2 mm
wide, but nearly 2 cm high. This resulting peculiar shape increases resistance to
flow, and as well very effectively allows larger particles ($>10\mu$) to impact on its
walls. The great surface area is remarkably effective in its abilities to warm and
humidify the entering air. This is explained by the extensive vascularization of
this tissue lining in the form of venous plexuses. The regulation of blood supply

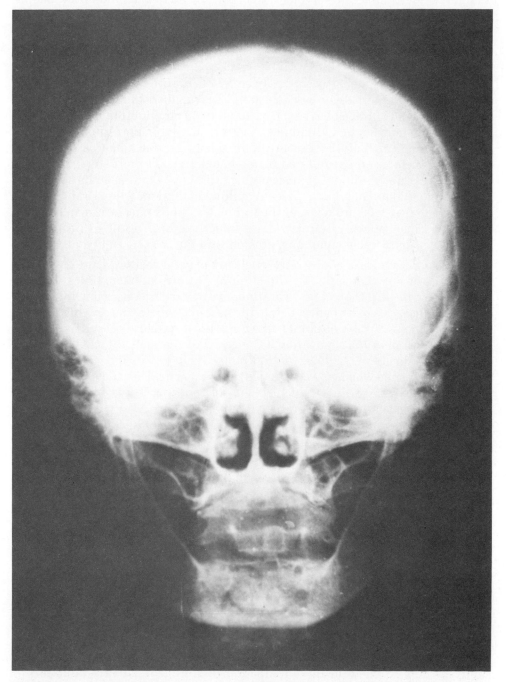

Figure 2-2.   X-ray illustration in the frontal plane to identify the two irregularly shaped nasal cavities separated by a median cartilaginous septum. Outlines of the frontal and orbital sinuses are also visible.

is largely under autonomic nervous system control. Increased blood flow (occurring with vasodilation) can compromise air flow by production of tissue edema. This accounts for the use of topically applied nasal medication (nose drops) to relieve congestion (by initiating vasoconstriction) and improve airflow dynamics.

Secretions empty into the nasal cavity both from the eye (via the lacrimal duct) and from the *paranasal sinuses*. There are a large number of these sinuses, or air cells, with a total volume of as much as 40 ml to 60 ml, differing in size, shape, and exact location among individuals. They are located in the ethmoid, frontal, sphenoid, and maxillary bones, and their names are the same as the bones containing them. Sinuses are lined by a ciliated mucus membrane which produces a rather watery fluid. Drainage of this fluid must occur at a rate similar to its rate of production in order to prevent buildup of fluid pressure. Drainage into the nasal cavity occurs from under the turbinates. Sinus infections can occur if drainage is inadequate. Clinically, these infections may result in headaches, abscesses, or in extreme situations, erosion into the intracranial cavity.

The *nasopharynx* is at almost a 90° angle to the nasal cavity *(Figure 2-1)*. This results in a major change in the direction of airflow and sometimes poses a challenge for the insertion of tubes destined for the trachea or stomach. The two aspects of the nasal cavity converge into the nasopharynx via narrowings termed the *internal nares*. From this point to the lungs the respiratory passage is a single tube. The term *pharynx* stems from a Greek word meaning "throat." The nasal portion extends to the region of the *soft palate*, with its appendage, the *uvula*. The uvula is visible when viewed through the oral cavity. The palate is the roof of the mouth and has two components. The soft portion differs from the more anterior hard palate in having no bony support.

At the origin of the nasopharynx, it is the posterior wall that receives the greatest impaction of inhaled foreign particulate material as air suddenly changes its direction of flow. Hence, it is appropriate that lymphatic tissue be located in the posterior wall of this area to permit interaction with this foreign material. There are 2 *pharyngeal tonsils*, and the term *adenoids* refers to their hypertrophy (enlargement), seen quite often among children. Because their expansion can significantly interfere with nasal breathing, adenoidectomy is sometimes performed.

In this same region of the nasopharynx appear the openings for the 2 *eustachian tubes*, also called *auditory tubes*, which connect the nasopharynx to the middle ear. These tubes allow equalization of pressure between the middle ear space and the atmosphere. The tubes are normally closed. Generation of tension in two muscles, the dilator tubae and salpingopharyngeus, results in opening of the eustachian or auditory tubes. This occurs during swallowing. Oftentimes, children ascending in elevators or airplanes are given a piece of candy or gum to chew in the anticipation of sufficient saliva production to promote swallowing, thereby assisting in equalization of atmospheric and middle ear pressures. Mucosal congestion, excessive sinus drainage, and overgrown adenoid tissue all impair normal eustachian or auditory tube operation.

The *oropharynx*, often referred to as the throat, comprises the region below the nasopharynx, above the laryngopharynx, and posterior to the oral (mouth) cavity. It is readily seen by looking into the mouth towards its posterior wall. The term *fauces* refers to the opening from the mouth into the oropharynx. In this region another group of tonsils, called faucial or *palatine tonsils*, are located. It is the palatine tonsils that are most often removed by a tonsillectomy as a result of enlargement. A third group, the lingual tonsils, are in this same general region, at the base of the tongue.

The largest structure in the oral cavity is the tongue. It extends into the oropharynx and under certain circumstances can block air flow into the lower respiratory tract. The tongue's posterior surface is well innervated. The appropriate receptor endings can initiate protective gagging reflexes. Even light pressure, by a finger or a medical instrument such as a tongue depressor, can trigger a gag response.

LARYNX AND TRACHEA

The *larynx* is an exceptionally complex and intricate series of cartilages connected to bones by muscles. It is commonly called the "voice box" because of its modification for speech; this does not impede the flow of air. It is often termed the "watchdog" of the lung. Its primary function has evolved to prevent the contamination of the lower respiratory tract with swallowed material destined for the gastrointestinal system. Should anything but air enter the trachea via the larynx, coughing ensues, with laryngeal constriction. Drowning victims usually have very little water in their lungs, succumbing to asphyxiation as a result of laryngeal spasm. It is only sometime following death that relaxation of the skeletal muscles protecting the airway permits the water to enter, assuming the victim has remained submerged.

The region of the larynx and esophagus forms a crucial crossroads. There has been speculation, notably by Wallace Fenn, on the significance of such an arrangement. Food should never be present in the respiratory tract, so why should the esophageal opening be so close to the airway? We do not need air in the gastrointestinal tract, so why should the larynx be so close with a tightly closed hypopharyngeal sphincter at the entrance to the esophagus to keep air out? The explanation may be that in other species the specialization of the pharynx for speech is much reduced, and the larynx and epiglottis are positioned higher in the respiratory tract.

There are three paired cartilages, three unpaired cartilages, eight pairs of extrinsic muscles, and five pairs of intrinsic muscles in the larynx, all held together by an equally impressive assortment of bones and ligaments. Various of these structures are involved with swallowing, prevention of food entry into the trachea, and phonation.

Of the three unpaired cartilages, the leaf-shaped *epiglottis* is the only one occasionally visible from the mouth *(Figure 2-1)*. It is often seen in crying infants. Located at the base of the tongue close to the oropharynx, the epiglottis is the chief guardian of the laryngeal opening.

The *cricoid cartilage* is the only complete cartilaginous ring in the entire larynx and trachea *(Figure 2-3)*. It is at the level of the sixth cervical vertebra. The cricoid is located below the Adam's apple, which is really the prominence of the *thyroid cartilage*, the largest of all the laryngeal cartilages. In part the cricoid cartilage is covered by the thyroid gland *(Figure 2-4)*. This gland has two lobes connected by an isthmus which covers the ventral cricoid prominence. An emergency surgical cricothyrotomy can be performed by an incision through the small space separating the cricoid and thyroid cartilages anteriorly. In contrast, a surgical tracheostomy is performed about 3 cm below the cricoid cartilage *(Figure 2-4)*. After the initial incision, the thyroid isthmus is divided and separated, and then a small window is created in the trachea for placement of a tracheostomy tube.

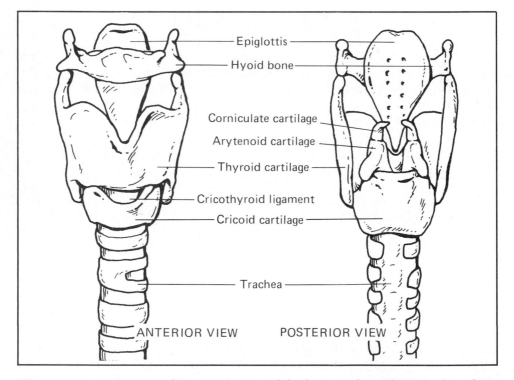

Figure 2-3.   Anterior and posterior view of the laryngeal cartilages and trachea.

The three paired cartilages are the *arytenoid, corniculate,* and *cuneiform* *(Figure 2-3)*. The arytenoids are the most important, playing a role both in phonation and in glottis patency. Intrinsic muscles connect to these cartilages and aid in their function.

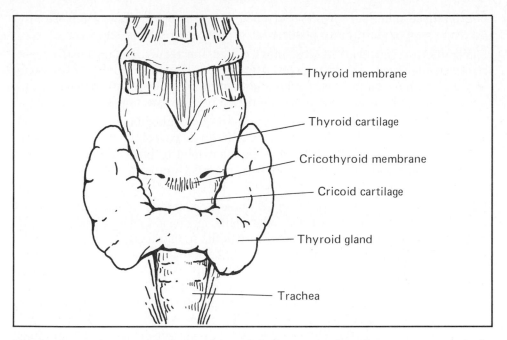

Thyroid membrane

Thyroid cartilage

Cricothyroid membrane

Cricoid cartilage

Thyroid gland

Trachea

Figure 2-4.   Anatomic relationships of the larynx and trachea as seen anteriorly to indicate the difference between two surgical procedures—cricothyrotomy and tracheostomy—performed to establish an emergency airway.

The vocal ligaments or cords attach to the arytenoid cartilages and then traverse the larynx to the thyroid cartilage. In this way the pitch of the voice is regulated. Women have vocal cords about 5 mm shorter than those of men; hence, their voice is initially pitched higher. Lateral rotation of the arytenoid cartilages by the posterior cricoarytenoideus muscle spreads the cords apart and at the same time opens the glottis. The opposite action—glottis closure and cord approximation—is accomplished by the lateral cricoarytenoideus. The true glottis is thus the space between the vocal cords.

The extrinsic muscles—omohyoids, sternohyoids, sternothyroids, thyrohyoids, stylopharyngeus, and palatopharyngeus—all connect to the various bones aiding in support of the larynx. The other sets of extrinsic muscles are sphincters in their activity, i.e., the inferior and superior constrictors.

In recent years many of the pharyngeal and laryngeal muscles have taken on added interest as physicians attempt to understand occurrences of asphyxia during sleep occasioned by upper airway obstruction. Two such situations are adult sleep apnea and sudden infant death syndrome. Ever since electromyographic evidence revealed a diminished upper airway muscle tone simultaneous with such obstruction during sleep, studies have been directed toward an understanding of how these muscles are activated or deactivated in response to stimuli that drive the diaphragm. Sleep brings with it clearly identifiable changes in the on-going respiratory rhythm. The extent to which unconsciousness modifies the tone of these other muscles is only beginning to be studied. Such exciting inquiries may explain these obstructive apneas seen during sleep.

The *inferior laryngeal nerves,* often called the recurrent laryngeal nerves, innervate all of the intrinsic muscles of the larynx. They are branches of the vagus nerves. Care must be exercised when performing a tracheostomy to ensure that these nerves, which lie on either side of the trachea, are not damaged.

The adult trachea *(Figure 2-5)* is an 11 cm to 13 cm tube placed half in the neck and half in the thorax. It is clearly not an anatomical part of the lung. Yet, it is the first part of the respiratory tract thus far described to have the air contained within it consistently and properly prepared (humidified, purified, and warmed) for entry into the lung.

The trachea has a series of 16 to 20 horseshoe-shaped cartilages embedded within its fibrous and smooth muscular walls, arranged laterally and ventrally, with the posterior wall composed entirely of the nonstriated *trachealis muscle.* *(Figure 2-5).* The rings help to prevent tubular collapse by increased thoracic pressure during a cough, although partial collapse does occur. During the inspiratory portion, such reduction of cross-sectional area increases gas velocity, and makes the cough effective. Tracheal collapse during this expiratory portion is not a threat, since the pressure through the trachea is supra-atmospheric. A real threat of tracheal collapse, however, can occur during the deep, rapid inspiratory portion. Thus, the cartilage rings are of great value.

The trachea is anchored caudally by a membrane connecting it to the pericardium and diaphragm. The tracheal dimensions change almost continuously because of postural movements of the head and neck, movements of the larynx and diaphragm, and a continually fluctuating intrathoracic pressure.

TRUNK STRUCTURES ASSOCIATED WITH BREATHING

The central part of the body is the trunk, and is continuous with the head, upper limbs, and lower limbs. The body wall is composed of the outer tissues of the trunk, and encloses the thoracic and abdominal cavities. These are normally filled with organs, blood vessels, nerves, and connective tissues. The *diaphragm* separates the two cavities. It is a dome-shaped musculo-tendinous sheet formed by muscle fibers originating in the body wall and inserting into a central tendon. This and other muscles functioning in breathing will be detailed in Chapter Three.

The *thoracic cavity* above the diaphragm and the *abdominal cavity* below the diaphragm comprise the two descriptive areas of the trunk known as the thorax and abdomen *(Figure 2-6).* The thorax is cone-shaped. It must be rigid to protect the vital organs; hence, part of it is bone and cartilage. But, it must also be resilient and have the ability to expand and reduce its volume. Normally, (subatmospheric) pressures exist in the thoracic cavity. Hence, to keep the thorax from

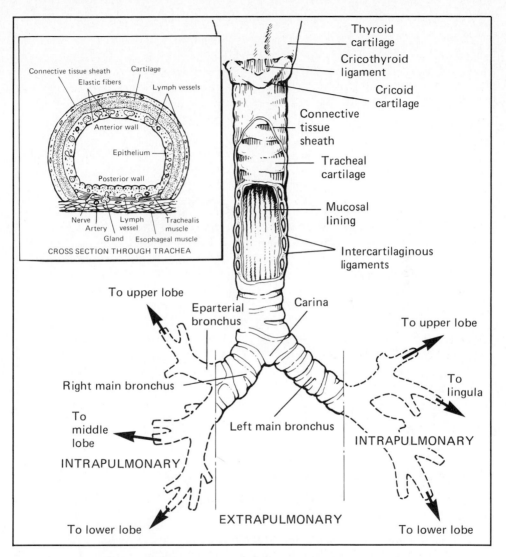

Figure 2-5. Anterior view of the trachea and primary bronchi, and a cross-section through a part of the trachea including a c-shaped cartilaginous element. This cartilage is not a completely encircling ring, with the trachealis muscle providing the necessary protective support posteriorly.

collapsing, its muscular walls are reinforced laterally and anteriorly by bones. The *sternum*, or breastbone, is a large flat bone in the anterior wall. Its adult form is composed of three parts. The *manubrium* is uppermost, the *body* forms the middle portion, and the *xiphoid process* is at the lower end. The lateral edges are the articulation points for the cartilages of the upper 7 ribs.

The *ribs* (or *costae*) are long curved bones extending from the vertebral column to form part of the chest wall. Between the ribs are the internal and external

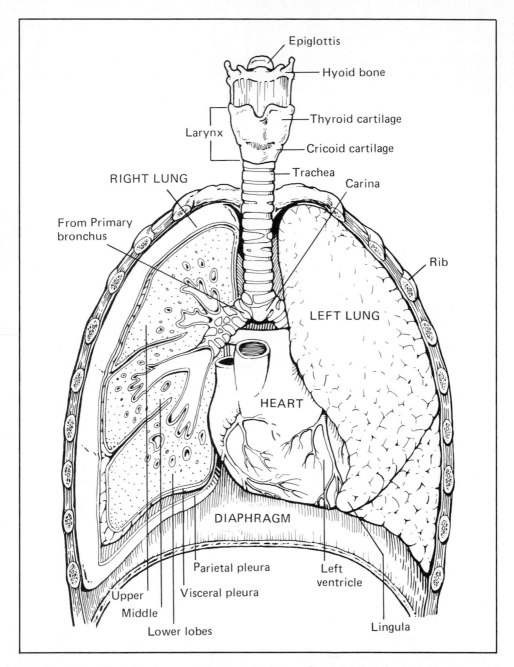

Figure 2-6.   Sketch of gross anatomic relationships in the thoracic cavity and mediastinum, as seen anteriorly with ribs and sternum removed. Redrawn with permission from *Scientific American* 202 (1): p. 139, Scientific American, Inc.: New York, 1960.

intercostal muscles. Intercostal nerves, arteries, and veins also course through this region. The first nine pairs of ribs articulate posteriorly with two vertebral bodies and also to the transverse process of the lower vertebra. The 10th pair articulates with only one vertebra—its body and transverse process. The lowermost ribs articulate only with a single vertebral body. All ribs are continued anteriorly with cartilage. The 10 upper pairs of ribs attach to the sternum by this cartilage; seven pairs each directly (true ribs), and the lower three pairs indirectly via the cartilage above (false ribs). The lower two pairs do not attach, and are often called floating ribs. The cartilage serves to enhance greatly the elasticity of the chest as it expands and recoils during breathing.

Anatomical similarities of all the ribs include 1) a *head, neck,* and *tubercle* on the posterior or vertebral end, 2) an *angle,* and 3) a *body* or *shaft (Figure 2-7)*. The first rib is very much curved, being the shortest, and has only slight motion. Ribs 2 through 7 become progressively longer, and are very important in ventilation.

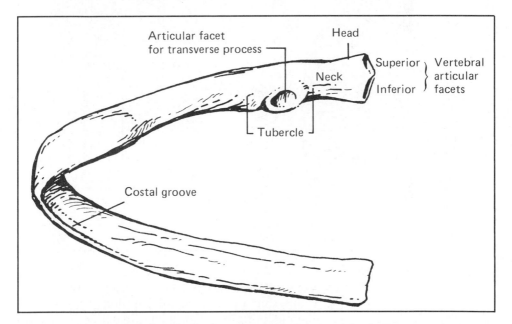

Figure 2-7.   A typical middle rib, from the left side of the body, viewed posteriorly (from the back). The head end (and tubercle) articulate with the vertebral column, while the shaft articulates with the sternum.

Ribs 8 through 12 become progressively shorter in length. These ribs move in somewhat similar fashion to those just described, particularly ribs 8 through 10, and only the transverse dimension of the chest changes. Elevation of the anterior ends of these ribs decreases the anterio-posterior diameter because the caudal end of the sternum is pulled toward the vertebral column.

During inspiration and expiration the ribs undergo simultaneous movement about two axes such that both the anterioposterior and transverse diameters of the thoracic cavity are increased. Movement about the axis extending from the tubercle through the sternum produces an effect much like raising a bucket handle, and changes the transverse diameter of the chest *(Figure 2-8B)*. Rotation about the axis extending through the head, neck and tubercle leads to a movement resembling the motion of a pump handle, thereby altering the anterioposterior diameter *(Figure 2-8C)*. Both of these movements, of course, occur simultaneously during breathing, and the volume of the chest is varied considerably. People who engage in long periods of very deep breathing, seen for example among athletes who train intensively for competitive swimming, may gradually develop an enlarged thorax. The ribs may assume a position that is more horizontal than usually seen, and greater lung volumes can result.

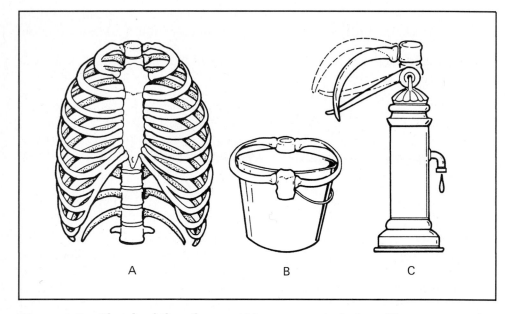

A   B   C

Figure 2-8.   Sketch of the rib cage (A) as seen anteriorly, with accompanying illustrations that diagram the two axes of rib movement; one about the rib tubercle through the sternum imitating a bucket-handle motion (B), the other through the head, neck, and tubercle imitating a pump handle (C). Figures B & C redrawn with permission from *Handbook of Physiology* Section 3, *Respiration I*, p. 234, American Physiological Society: Washington, 1964.

The thoracic cavity includes the lungs, heart, esophagus, and other associated structures *(Figure 2-6)*. The center of this cavity is the *mediastinum*, a term literally meaning "place in the middle." The region is diverse and contains parts of the trachea and esophagus, portions of large blood vessels entering and leaving the heart, the thoracic duct, lymph nodes, remains of the thymus gland, and many nerves, including the phrenic and vagus.

On each side of the mediastinum are two serous fluid-containing cavities—the *pleural cavities.* The lungs are invaginated into their medial walls in a manner similar to fists pressed into the sides of balloons. When the thorax expands during inspiration, the pleural cavities expand. The outer parietal pleura lines the chest wall and expands with inspiration. Because the inner visceral pleura is attached to the lungs, it expands as well. The thin residual film of fluid in the pleural cavities provides lubrication for the sliding of the visceral pleura on the parietal pleura with each breath.

THE LUNGS

The lungs are not identical in size. The heart and pericardium bulge more into the left side of the thorax *(Figure 2-6)* than into the right. Also, the right portion of the diaphragm, which is directly above the liver, is higher than the left. Both lungs are divided into *lobes* by fissures lined with visceral pleura penetrating into the actual lung substance. The right lung has an upper, middle and lower lobe, whereas the left lung has an upper and lower lobe, with an appendage of the upper lobe known as the *lingula (Figure 2-6).* The *root* or *hilum* of each lung is in the center of its medial surface. Here the bronchi, arteries, nerves and veins enter and leave the lung, respectively, via the mediastinum. At rest, the root of each lung is behind a line joining the sternal ends of the second and fourth costal cartilages.

The trachea bifurcates into *primary bronchi* at the level of the aortic arch and the fifth thoracic vertebra. A cartilaginous septum (or spur to the bronchoscopist) just to the left of the midline at the base of this bifurcation is called the *carina.* It thus preferentially directs air flow more toward the right bronchus. The left primary bronchus is slightly smaller than the right, and angles more sharply toward its intended lung, at 45° to 55° from the midline, passing immediately in front of the esophagus. This inclination reduces the incidence of aspiration of an object into that bronchus. By contrast, the larger right bronchus angles only at 20° to 30° from the midline, dividing into branches passing above and below the pulmonary artery and then entering the lung. The most common site of aspiration for lodged objects is in the right lower lobes of the lung.

A most crucial aspect of pulmonary anatomy is that the larger branches of the bronchi supply very discrete portions of lung tissue that match precisely the lobes and segments. This is a function of embryological development. Understanding this three-dimensional arrangement permits a better appreciation for the importance of bronchial obstruction in the lobe or segment ventilated by it. Each *bronchopulmonary segment* has a specific name, as illustrated in *Figure 2-9.*

The *bronchi* divide repeatedly within the lungs to form an inverted tree-like arrangement of tubes for ventilation. These, as well as the trachea, contain regularly arranged horseshoe-shaped elements of cartilage in their walls, becoming gradually more developed in the trachea and irregular and less complete in

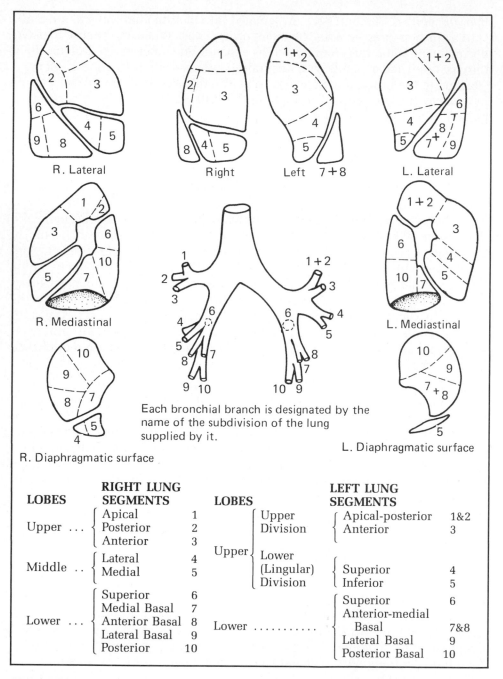

Each bronchial branch is designated by the name of the subdivision of the lung supplied by it.

R. Lateral

Right   Left 7+8

L. Lateral

R. Mediastinal

L. Mediastinal

R. Diaphragmatic surface

L. Diaphragmatic surface

LOBES	RIGHT LUNG SEGMENTS		LOBES	LEFT LUNG SEGMENTS	
Upper ...	Apical	1	Upper Division	Apical-posterior	1&2
	Posterior	2		Anterior	3
	Anterior	3			
Middle ..	Lateral	4	Upper — Lower (Lingular) Division	Superior	4
	Medial	5		Inferior	5
Lower ...	Superior	6	Lower	Superior	6
	Medial Basal	7		Anterior-medial Basal	7&8
	Anterior Basal	8		Lateral Basal	9
	Lateral Basal	9		Posterior Basal	10
	Posterior	10			

Figure 2-9 Bronchopulmonary segments of the human lung as viewed from several surfaces. Redrawn with permission from Jackson, C.L. and Huber, J.F., *Diseases of the Chest* 9:324, 1943.

the bronchi. The cartilage remains only as cartilaginous plates in the segmental bronchi. The first generation of tubes not to have cartilages are termed *bronchioles*.

Each mainstream bronchus divides more than 20 times *(Figure 2-10)*, as shown by the detailed studies of Ewald Weibel. Only during the terminal 8 divisions (or generations) does any gas exchange occur with the blood. This region is thus often termed the *respiratory zone* to distinguish it from the *conducting zone* above. Generally these divisions (bronchial or bronchiolar) are dichotomous, i.e., each divides into two daughter bronchi or bronchioles of approximately equal diameters. Each division results in an increase of airway cross sectional area of about 20% from that of the parent airway. The bronchioles eventually

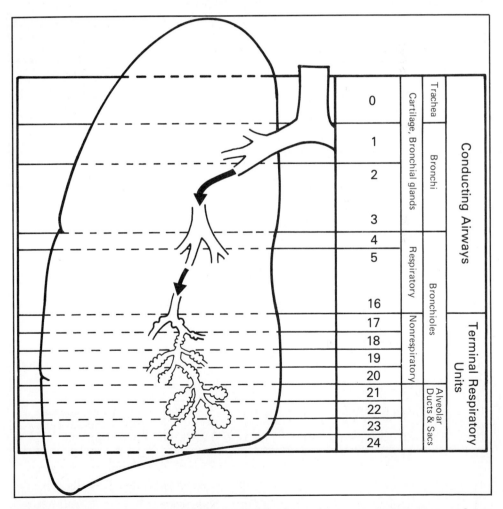

Figure 2-10.   Generations (divisions) of the branching respiratory tree as elucidated through the research of Ewald Weibel. Adapted from Weibel, E., *Morphometry of the Human Lung*, p. 111, Springer-Verlag: Berlin, 1973.

divide further into *alveolar ducts* and *sacs*, each containing dozens of individual *alveoli*.

Curiously, the size of the daughter airway is related to the relative angle that it takes from the longitudinal direction of the airway. If each leaves at an equal angle, then the respective diameters are approximately the same. When the angles of progression differ substantially, the airway deviating most from the main line of the parent has the smallest diameter. This pattern is nearly ideal for equal distribution of inspired air through the lungs. When the distance from any parent airway to the lung periphery is short, small branches from the parent bronchus spiral outward laterally. The typical bronchus may branch 22 or more times; these lateral pathways have only 4 to 6 generations. Histological details of these airways will be discussed in Chapter Five.

TABLE 2-1.   Subdivisions of the Respiratory Tree*

Generation	Name	Diameter cm	Length cm	Number per generation	Histological Notes
0	Trachea	1.8	12	1	Wealth of goblet cells
1	Primary Bronchi	1.2	4.8	2	Right larger than left
2	Lobar Bronchi	0.8	0.9	5	3 right, 2 left
3	Segmental Bronchi	0.6	0.8	19	10 right; 8 left
4	Subsegmental Bronchi	0.5	1.3	20	
5 ↓ 10	Small Bronchi	0.4 / 0.1	1.1 / 0.5	40 / 1020	Still have cartilage; many cell types as well as respiratory epithelium
11 ↓ 13	Bronchioles Primary & Secondary	0.1 / 0.1	0.4 / 0.3	2050 / 8190	No cartilage; smooth muscle, cilia, goblet cells present
14 ↓ 15	Terminal Bronchioles	0.1 / 0.1	0.2 / 0.2	16380 / 32770	No goblet cells; smooth muscle, cilia, and cuboidal cells
16 ↓ 18	Respiratory Bronchioles	0.1 / 0.1	0.2 / 0.1	65540 / 262140	No smooth muscle; cilia, cuboidal cells; cilia disappear
19 ↓ 23	Alveolar Ducts	0.05 / 0.04	0.1 / 0.05	524290 / 8390000	No cilia; cuboidal cells
24	Alveoli+	244	238	300000000	

*Adapted from E.R. Weibel, *Morphometry of the Human Lung*, Springer Verlag: Berlin, 1973.
+Alveolar dimensions given in micrometers.

All of the blood output of the right ventricle is transported to the lungs via the large pulmonary artery. This vessel promptly divides into right and left pulmonary arteries that enter the hilum of each lung. The pulmonary arterial tree accompanies the bronchial tree, dividing as the latter divides. About 30% of the total pulmonary blood volume is in the arteries; 60% is in the veins and 20% is in the capillaries.

The walls of the pulmonary artery branches are composed principally of elastic tissue. The blood vessel walls in the region of the bronchioles contain vascular smooth muscle, but this muscular layer is very thin relative to that found in other vascular beds. At the level of the terminal bronchioles the arteries have a diameter of about 100 μm. Beyond the terminal bronchioles the arterial tree subdivides into arterioles with walls composed primarily of elastic connective tissue. Smooth muscle is also present at this level, but the muscle fibers appear discontinuous. The arterioles break up into a capillary network that essentially provides a pool of mixed venous (i.e., poorly oxygenated) blood surrounding the alveoli *(Figure 2-11)*.

The dynamics of capillary blood flow in the lungs are impressive. If we assume a cardiac output of 4900 ml/min, and a pulmonary capillary blood volume of 70 ml, then this capillary blood will be replaced 70 times each minute during resting conditions! During exercise the pulmonary capillary bed will be expanded enormously and these flow dynamics will also increase.

If fresh water enters the alveoli it will very rapidly move into the pulmonary circulation. It moves down its osmotic gradient. This same gradient prevents transudation of fluid into the alveoli from the bloodstream. The osmotic pressure of the circulating plasma proteins (tending to bring water into the circulation) ranges from 25 mmHg to 30 mmHG (3.3 to 4.0 kPa), whereas the pulmonary capillary pressure (tending to force fluid out of the circulation) is only about 7 mmHg (0.9 kPa). Thus, the pressure gradients serving, respectively, to promote fluid flow from an alveolus to the circulation and from the circulation to an alveolus are much greater in the former direction than in the latter. This demonstrates the importance of the low perfusion pressure prevalent in the pulmonary circulation. Serious problems could arise if the perfusion pressure became elevated. Most important would be an accumulation of fluid in the lungs. This condition is called pulmonary edema.

The *venous system* arises distal to the alveolocapillary network. The arrangement of the venules is different from that of the arterioles. Venules collect into venous plexuses that lie in the interlobular septa. The pulmonary veins do not accompany the pulmonary arterial tree. They have direct connections to the supporting connective tissue, and their diameter is partially dependent upon tissue tension and lung volume.

Although the nutritional needs of the lung tissues are partly provided for by mixed venous blood, a smaller circulation comprised of highly oxygenated blood also assists in this regard. There is a separate *bronchial circulation* branching directly from the aorta, or from the intercostal, subclavian, or internal mammary arteries. Lung transplant patients do not require bronchial arteries for

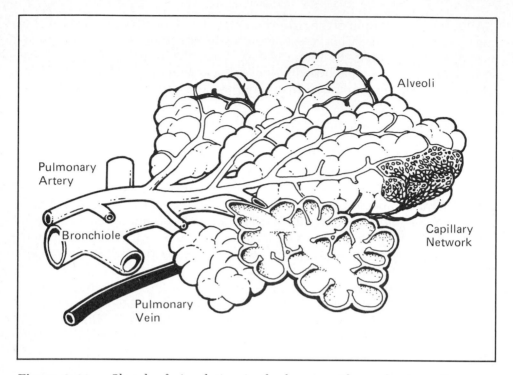

Figure 2-11.   Sketch of circulation in the lungs, with emphasis on the enormous expansion of the capillary network in the alveolar regions to ensure efficient gas exchange between alveolar air and pulmonary capillary blood. Reprinted with permission from *Scientific American* 207 (1): p. 139, Scientific American, Inc.: New York, 1962.

pulmonary survival, hence this circulation in the adult lung is supplementary. The bronchial arteries course along the dorsal wall of each primary bronchus and supply the bronchial walls to the level of terminal bronchioles. At this level, the bronchial arterial supply breaks into plexuses, some of which anastomose with capillaries from the pulmonary arteries and eventually drain into the pulmonary venous system. Being poorly oxygenated, this blood mixes with freshly arterialized blood and reduces slightly its O_2 content. This concept of physiologic shunting of blood will be discussed in detail in Chapter Eight. The majority of the bronchial circulation empties into the azygos vein, enroute to the superior vena cava and the right heart. There is an asymmetry here in that the right bronchial vein empties directly into the azygos vein, whereas the left bronchial vein empties first into either the left intercostal or accessory hemiazygos veins *(Figure 2-12)*.

The lungs are more richly supplied with *lymphatic tissue* than any other organ. Perhaps this is related to the enormous exposure of the lungs to the external environment. Lymphatic vessels are present wherever there is loose connective tissue within the lung parenchyma. They parallel much of the vas-

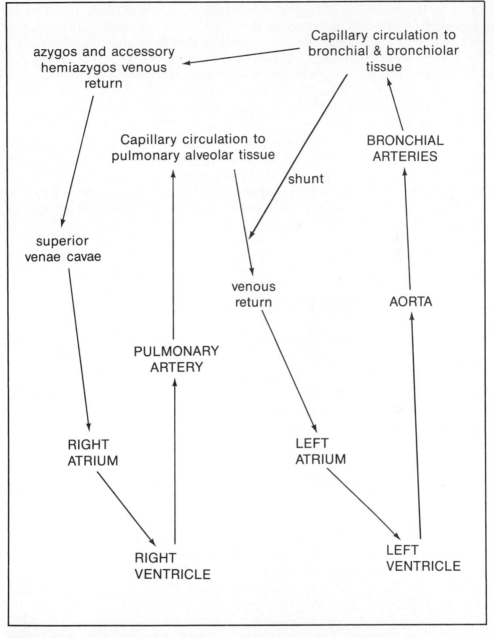

Figure 2-12. Flow diagram illustrating general aspects of the pulmonary and bronchial circulations, showing how shunting of some venous blood from the bronchial circulation into the oxygenated blood of the pulmonary vein can occur normally.

culature. The vessels are delicate and collapsible, and are subject to alteration by changes in intrapleural pressures. Lymph channels are supplied with tiny valves that ensure unidirectional flow. The distance from any alveolus to a lymph channel is very small. Aggregations of lymphoid tissue are present along respiratory bronchioles, other bronchioles, and bronchi, and are quite prominent at points of airway branching. The efferent flow of lymph, away from alveoli, is generally in the direction of the hilum. In addition, the pleural tissue has an extensive lymphatic system.

Despite this important lymphatic provision, the actual lymphatic drainage is not as large as one might initially imagine. The mean pulmonary arterial pressure is about 14 mmHg (1.0 kPa) and the left arterial pressure is about 5 mmHg (0.7 kPa). In between, the pulmonary capillary pressure will average about 7 mmHg (0.9 kPa). This is sufficiently low that leakage (extravasation) into the pulmonary lymphatic space is minimal.

RELEVANT READING

Andrew, B. The respiratory displacement of the larynx: a study of the accessory respiratory muscles. *Journal of Physiology* (Lond.) **130**: 474–487, 1955.

Chernick, N.S. Respiratory dysrhythmias in sleep. *New England Journal of Medicine*, **305**: 325–330, 1981.

Comroe, J. The Lung. *Scientific American* **214** (2): 56–58, 1966.

Dahl, D. Anatomy of the respiratory system. In *Egan's Fundamentals of Respiratory Therapy*. (C.B. Spearman, R.L. Sheldon, D.F. Egan, eds.), (C.V. Mosby Co., pp. 81–114), 1982.

Davies, P. The structure of respiratory defense mechanisms. *Seminars in Respiratory Medicine* **3**: 211–222, 1980.

Fenn, W.O. Perspective in phonation. *Annals of the New York Academy of Sciences*, **155**: 4–8, 1968.

Green, J.M., and Neil, E. The respiratory function of the laryngeal muscles. *Journal of Physiology* (Lond.) **129**: 134–139, 1955.

Moss, M.L. Veloepiglottic sphincter and obligate nose breathing in the neonate. *Journal of Pediatrics* **67**: 330–331, 1965.

Murray, J.F. *The Normal Lung*, W.B. Saunders Co., Philadelphia, 334 p., 1976.

Phillipson, E.A. Regulation of breathing during sleep. *American Review of Respiratory Disease* **115**: 217–227, 1977.

Proctor, D.F. The upper airways. I. Nasal physiology and defense of the lungs. *American Review of Respiratory Disease* **115**: 97–130, 1977.

Proctor, D.F. The upper airways. II. The larynx and trachea. *American Review of Respiratory Disease* **115**: 315–342, 1977.

Strohl, K.P. Upper airway muscles of respiration. *American Review of Respiratory Disease* **124:** 211–213, 1981.

Tenney, S.M. and Bartlett, D. Some comparative aspects of the control of breathing. In *Regulation of Breathing*, Part I (T.F. Hornbein, ed.), Marcel Dekker: New York, pp. 67–104, 1981.

Weibel, E. *Morphometry of the Human Lung.* Springer Verlag, Berlin, 1973.

Weibel, E. *The Pathway for Oxygen.* Harvard University Press, Cambridge, MA, 1984.

The Muscles of Breathing

Chapter Three

Chapter Three Outline

Supplying O_2 to alveoli and removing CO_2 from them is accomplished by the flow of air in and out of the lungs with each breath. To create the forces that produce inspiration and expiration, muscles are used and work is done. Resistance to the flow of air occurs because of 1) the elastic recoil of the lungs and thorax, 2) the frictional resistance caused by deformation of the tissues of the lungs and thorax, and 3) the frictional resistance from air flow through the many small tubes of the conducting airway. Muscles attempt to overcome these resistances. When the respiratory muscles are at rest, the thorax assumes the position of passive expiration. There is a balance between the outward expansion of the chest and the elastic recoil of the lungs. This position is termed the resting end-expiratory position, and the quantity of air contained within the lungs is called the functional residual capacity. Deviations from this position are produced through activation of the respiratory muscles. As respiration increases in terms of air volume moved per unit time, the number of muscles involved also increases. Aside from the heart, it would be difficult to find muscles with a more important function than the muscles of breathing. If ventilation fails, death is as sure as if the heart beat fails.

The respiratory muscles have no inherent rhythm, but rather generate tension as a result of a rhythmic pattern of neuron-induced action potentials activating them. Nerve cells that have a regulating influence on breathing originate in the respiratory centers located in the pons and medulla of the brainstem, though some may come from higher cortical areas. *(Figure 3-1)*. These neurons extend caudally as part of the lateral and anterior columns of the spinal cord, synapsing on anterior (ventral) horn cells. The axons of these anterior horn cells then continue into the periphery and terminate on the motor end plates of all the various skeletal muscle fibers which play a role in breathing.

THE DIAPHRAGM

The diaphragm is often considered as a muscle, but in fact is a dome-shaped musculo-fibrous septum separating the thoracic and abdominal cavities *(Figure 3-2)*. It does indeed have muscular fibers, and these form its periphery. Some of these fibers arise anteriorly from the xiphoid process of the sternum. Others arise laterally from the lower 6 ribs on either side. Additional fibers arise posteriorly from the lumbar vertebrae. They all converge and insert into a thin but strong central tendon to which the pericardium is attached. Its convex upper surface forms the floor of the thoracic cavity and its concave lower surface forms the roof of the abdominal cavity. This shape is caused in part by the elastic recoil of the lungs. The diaphragm has a surface area of approximately 250 cm^2, and the reduced intrathoracic pressure tends to pull it into the chest cavity. The diaphragm has several apertures, to permit such structures as the esophagus, aorta, inferior vena cava, and several visceral nerves to pass through.

The innervation of the muscular aspects of the diaphragm is by the phrenic nerve from the cervical plexus. Primarily, the fourth cervical nerve contributes to

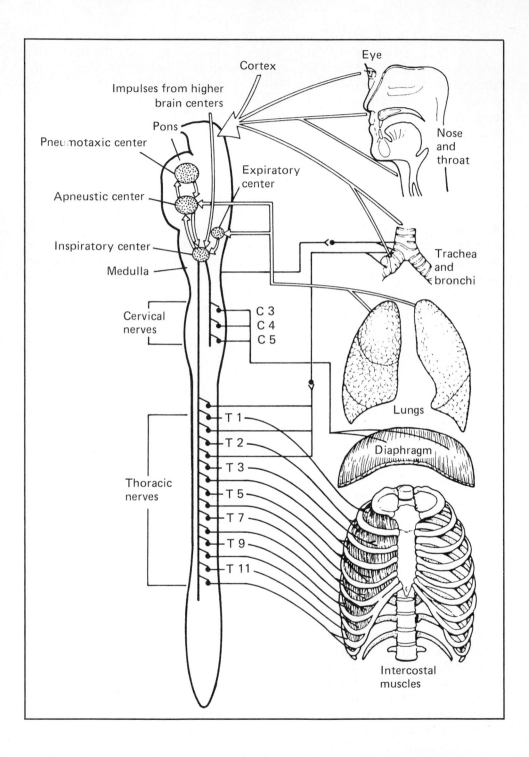

this plexus, with secondary contributions by the third and fifth cervical nerves (Figure 3-1). This explains why cervical spinal cord injury involving trauma to the C_3, C_4, and C_5 levels brings respiratory complications in addition to the other complex aspects of neurophysiologic disruption in such patients. It should be realized, however, that a supplemental innervation of the diaphragm by lower thoracic nerves can permit, with proper though time-consuming training, a gradual restoration of diaphragm function.

The result of tension generation by the diaphragm's muscular fibers is to draw its central tendon downward. This has two consequences. First, it increases thoracic volume, thereby lowering intrathoracic pressure. Second, it decreases the abdominal volume, thereby increasing intra-abdominal pressure. The dome of the diaphragm moves downward and somewhat forward, forcing the abdominal viscera downward as well; the abdominal wall tends to protrude. Two dimensions of the thoracic cavity are increased. The flattening of the diaphragm most noticeably increases the vertical dimension. The raising and eversion of the costal margin pulls it upward and outward, thereby increasing the transverse dimension. This is an important clinical point, since in situations where the diaphragm is abnormally low and relatively flat as in pulmonary emphysema, the vertical dimension will not be increased as much, but in addition the costal margin will be pulled inward, actually reducing the transverse dimension.

Although the diaphragm is a single anatomic structure, the union of its central tendon with the fibrous pericardium functionally divides the dome into 2 hemidiaphragms. At the end of a normal exhalation, i.e., in the resting end-expiratory position, the right dome, with the liver immediately below it, is about 1.5 cm higher than the left in 90% of the population. The movements of both hemidiaphragms are usually synchronous, even though each has its own nerve supply. Each may function independently of the other if one of the phrenic nerves becomes non-functional.

Figure 3-1.   Sketch of the various nervous connections between the central nervous system and the respiratory system. The driving mechanism for breathing resides in the pons and medulla of the brainstem. This rhythm can be altered voluntarily by input from the cerebral cortex. Stimuli from these brainstem centers influence the various muscles of breathing through connections involving the spinal cord (cervical and thoracic nerves). As inspiration occurs, stretching of tissues in and around the lungs sends inhibitory information back to these brainstem centers, mediating cessation of inspiration.

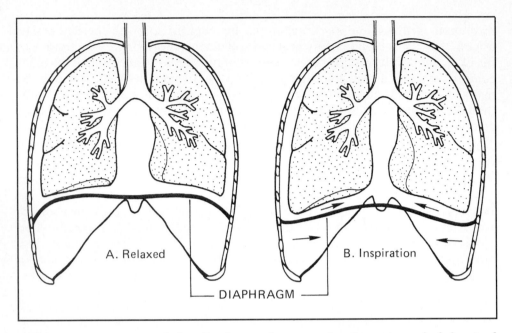

Figure 3-2. Position of the diaphragm between the thoracic and abdominal cavities A) before inspiration begins, i.e., at the end-expiratory position, and B) as it generates tension upon inspiration and descends, thereby increasing thoracic cavity volume and reducing its lower diameter. Redrawn with permission from *Egan's Fundamentals of Respiratory Therapy* (C.B. Spearman & R.L. Sheldon, eds.), Ch. 4, p. 124, C.V. Mosby Company: St. Louis, 1982.

The diaphragm moves downward about 1.25 cm during quiet breathing, and a 1 cm excursion approximates a 350 ml increase in volume. Thus, a normal excursion would result in the movement of about 440 ml of air—very nearly the normal tidal volume. During very intense exercise this downward diaphragm excursion may exceed 10 cm. Because of this volume relationship, and because of the long-standing knowledge that the diaphragm does generate tension during inspiration in healthy human subjects, the suggestion is often made that the diaphragm is the only active inspiratory muscle during the normal resting state. This is untrue. There is electromyographic evidence that the external intercostal muscles are active as well during inspiration. However, these intercostal muscles produce very little thoracic volume changes in comparison to the diaphragm. Those individuals who naturally utilize their diaphragm more than a combination of the diaphragm and intercostal muscles during resting breathing have a greater abdominal wall protrusion. When one is recumbent, the intercostal muscles assume a much greater role in generating the thoracic volume changes.

The position of the diaphragm in the thorax depends upon two main factors: 1) elasticity of the lung tissue, which tends to pull it upward, and 2) intra-abdominal tension caused by the abdominal muscles and volume of the abdominal viscera, which tends to push it upward. In a vertical (standing) position, the abdominal viscera cause a downward pull; these counteracting forces keep the diaphragm in a position intermediate to that found in the sitting and recumbent positions. When an individual is seated, the abdominal muscles are under much less tension. Thus, respiratory excursions are minimal in this position; it is here that severely dyspneic people find most comfort.

The statement is often made that the diaphragm is involved solely with ventilation. This is also incorrect. When the diaphragm actively generates tension at the same time as the abdominal muscles, this results in an increase in abdominal pressure which aids the abdominal viscera to discharge their contents, as in micturition, defecation, emesis, and parturition. The diaphragm in this same manner also facilitates coughing, sneezing, singing, and the playing of wind instruments. All of these involve abdominal muscle tension generation against a fixed diaphragm.

INTERCOSTAL MUSCLES

Controversy over the action of these muscles has been active ever since anatomical studies began, and because of the complexity of rib movements, their precise function has not been clearly elucidated. There are two planes of muscular and tendinous fibers that occupy each of the intercostal spaces (Figure 3-3). The external intercostal muscle fibers slope obliquely downward (inferiorly) and forward (anteriorly) from the rib above to the one below. They arise from the lower border of the rib above and insert into the upper border of the rib below. In humans there are 11 pairs of these.

Similarly, there are 11 pairs of internal intercostal muscles, which are beneath the external intercostals. They slope obliquely downward and posteriorly from the upper rib to the one below. They arise from the ridge on the inner surface of the rib above from its corresponding costal cartilage, and insert into the upper border of the rib below.

These muscles are all innervated by the intercostal nerves, which emerge from the first through eleventh thoracic spinal cord segments. During inspiration in quiet breathing the intercostal muscles generate tension and thus tend to keep the ribs in a constant position relative to one another. This gives stability to the chest wall. Electromyographic studies do not suggest a marked rhythmic increase and decrease in their activity that would imply a functional role in altering thoracic volume.

During increased breathing, as with exercise, such a rhythmic rise and fall in activity does occur. The first rib becomes fixed by the action of the scalene muscles. The external intercostal muscles, upon activation during inspiration, serve to lift the ribs by pulling them upward and outward, increasing the anteroposterior and transverse dimensions of the chest, thus expanding the

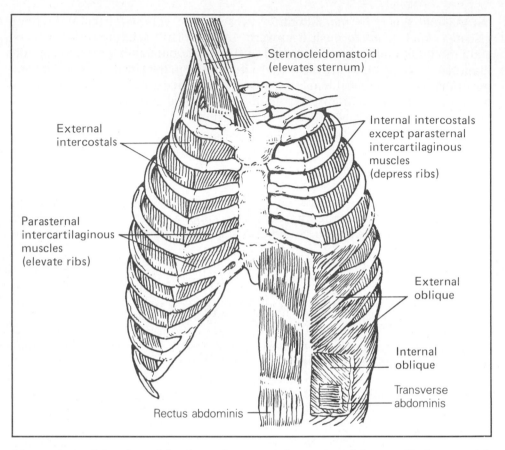

Figure 3-3.   Muscles of the thoracic cage and anterior abdomen. Redrawn with permission from Plate 5, Section I of *The Ciba Collection of Medical Illustrations*, Vol. 7, *Respiratory System*, p. 47, Ciba Pharmaceutical Company: Summit NJ, 1980.

thoracic volume. The portion of the internal intercostals between the rib cartilages also seems to elicit similar activity. The anatomic arrangement of the ribs is such that they are displaced upward more easily than downward. Recall the bucket handle and pump handle motion of the ribs, described in Chapter Two (Figure 2-8).

SCALENE MUSCLES

There are three pairs of scalene muscles, serving as important inspiratory muscles (Figure 3-4). The largest and longest is the scalenus medius. It arises from the posterior tubercles of the transverse processes of the third through sixth cervical vertebrae and also descends alongside the vertebral column to insert onto the first rib. The scalenus posterior is the smallest and deepest of the three and is difficult to observe on dissection. It arises from the transverse processes of the lower 2 or 3 cervical vertebrae and inserts onto the second rib. The innervation of these muscles is via the cervical nerves.

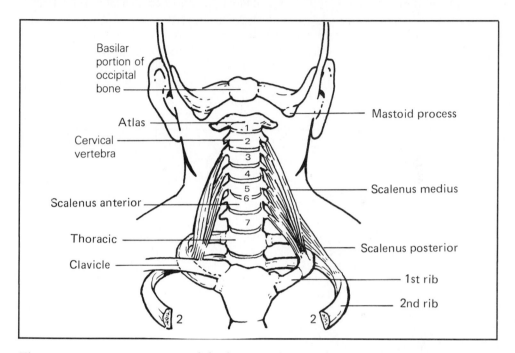

Figure 3-4.   Posterior view of the head and neck, showing vertebral bodies and attachments of the scalene muscles to these as well as to the first two ribs. Redrawn with permission from *Principles and Practice of Respiratory Therapy,* 2nd Ed., (J.A. Young and D. Crocker, eds.), p. 49, Year Book Medical Publishers, Inc.: Chicago, 1976.

These muscles can be better appreciated if one closes the glottis and then attempts an inspiration. This is a static inspiration since no airflow into the lungs will occur. As considerable effort is expended, reducing the intra-alveolar pressure markedly, the scaleni will be noticeable in their tension generation, and can easily be felt. Even during quiet breathing the scaleni demonstrate rhythmic electromyographic activity. Their action is to elevate the first and second ribs. During inspiration they help increase the thoracic volume, although the actual volume contribution is very small. Since quiet expiration is a passive process, these muscles display almost no electrical activity. They can be mobilized effectively to aid inspiration in both healthy exercising people and in patients with pulmonary disease. However, during these instances the scalene muscles also generate tension during expiration, and in coughing assist to prevent herniation of the apex of the lung between the ribs.

STERNOCLEIDOMASTOID MUSCLES

These rather large bilaterally arranged muscles elevate the sternum and increase the anteroposterior chest diameter during vigorous inspiration. They arise from the manubrium and medial clavicle, and insert into the mastoid process of the temporal bone *(Figure 3-5)*. The spinal accessory nerve (cranial nerve XI) and second cervical nerve supply them. They have no function in expiration. Patients with airway obstruction and hyperinflation use these even during resting breathing. In such cases, it is often possible to see these muscles actively generating tension and lifting the clavicle with each inspiration. Similarly, athletes involved in nearly maximal ventilatory efforts often have these visibly active.

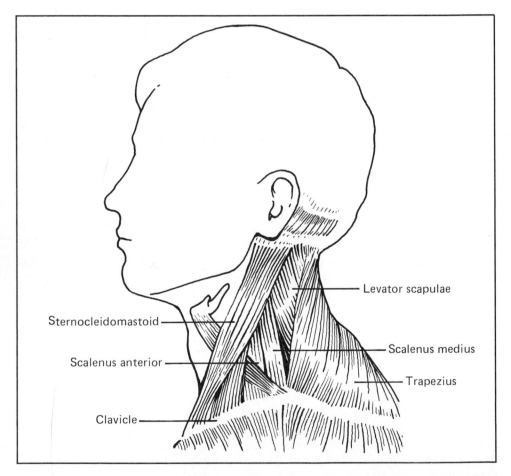

Figure 3-5. Lateral view of the accessory muscles of breathing found in the neck. Redrawn with permission from Fig. 433 of *Anatomy of the Human Body*, by Henry Gray, 27th ed. (C.M. Goss, ed.), p. 433, Lea & Febiger: Philadelphia, 1959.

ABDOMINAL MUSCLES

These are the most important muscles of expiration. They include the external obliques, the internal obliques, the transversus abdominis, and the rectus abdominis (Figure 3-3). All of them are supplied by the seventh through twelfth thoracic nerves and the first lumbar nerve. The action of these muscles, when they generate tension, is 1) a compression of the abdominal contents, 2) a flexion of the trunk, 3) an increase in intraabdominal pressure, and 4) a pulling of the lower ribs downward and medially.

When an individual is resting in the supine position, the abdominal muscles generate virtually no tension, but, as the standing posture is assumed, they become active. This tension is unrelated to the normal resting breathing cycle, and probably relates to the antigravity role of these muscles. It also has the effect of minimizing the increase in end-expiratory lung volume that would otherwise be more marked upon standing, caused by the downward traction of the abdominal viscera on the diaphragm.

Under normal conditions, in either the supine or erect position these muscles show little activity until ventilation increases to approximately 40 L/min (for example, 1,500 ml tidal volume × 26 breaths per minute = 40 L/m). However, during airflow obstruction these muscles may be activated early to assist expiration. By creating a strong, intra-abdominal pressure to drive the diaphragm like a piston into the thoracic cavity, a powerful generator of force is available to accomplish expiration. Patients with chronic obstructive pulmonary disease often have little effective use of these muscles and are at considerable disadvantage.

De Troyer has suggested very logically that active abdominal muscles can be thought of as accessory inspiratory muscles, for two reasons. One concerns the greater reduction in end-expiratory lung volume that occurs when abdominal muscle tension generation powerfully assists in emptying the lungs during increased breathing. As will be discussed further in Chapter Six, there is now greater elastic recoil in the respiratory system, making it easier for inflation to proceed. The other concerns the longer length of diaphragm muscle fibers at the start of any inspiration. This is caused by the previous expiration vigorously forcing the abdominal viscera toward the thorax. By lengthening the diaphragm muscle fibers, they are now able to generate optimum tension since there are an optimum number of cross-linkages between the actin and myosin molecules in the muscle cells.

PECTORALIS MAJOR

In patients with great air hunger it is as if all the muscles of the body sense the need for combining forces to coordinate and assist in breathing. Such an example is found in the pectoralis major (Figure 3-6). This is a powerful bilateral anterior chest muscle with the primary function of pulling the upper arms toward the midline in a hugging motion (flexing, adducting, and rotating). It is a large fan-shaped muscle arising from the medial half of the clavicle, the anterior surface of the sternum, the first 6 costal cartilages, and a fibrous sheath enclosing muscles of the abdominal wall. The muscle fibers converge into a thick tendon that inserts into the upper part of the humerus bone.

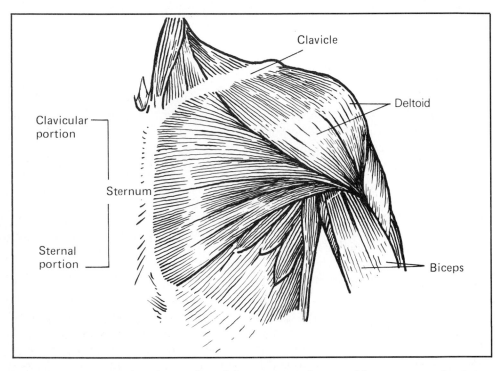

Figure 3-6.   Superficial muscles of the anterior chest and forearm, emphasizing the pectoralis major and deltoideus. Redrawn with permission from Fig. 457 of *The Anatomy of the Human Body*, by Henry Gray, 27th ed. (C.M. Goss, ed)., p. 489, Lea & Febiger: Philadelphia, 1959.

However, if the arms and shoulders are fixed, as by leaning on the elbows or firmly grasping the back of a chair or the end of a bed (the scapula will be fixed by tension generation in the levator scapulae, the trapezius, and the rhomboideus), then the pectoralis can use its normal insertion as an origin and pull with great force on the anterior chest, lifting up the ribs and sternum and increasing the thoracic anteroposterior diameter during inspiration. Patients with chronic obstructive pulmonary disease assume characteristic poses for maximum use of their pectoralis muscles. The serratus anterior also assists in this regard.

SUMMARY OF MUSCLE ACTIONS
IN HEALTHY BREATHING

During quiet inspiration the diaphragm generates tension, greatly increasing the vertical dimension of the thoracic cavity, as well as its transverse dimension. The first and second ribs remain fixed by the resistance of structures in the cervical region, caused in part by activation of the scaleni. The remaining ribs except the last two (floating ribs) are brought upward toward them by tension generated in the external intercostals. This upward rib motion increases the anteroposterior and transverse diameters of the thorax. Until recently quiet expiration has been considered a passive process, occurring as a result of a reduction in nervous stimulation to all muscles concerned with breathing. Recent work by Stephen Loring and Jere Mead suggests that even at rest, at least in the standing position, people do actively generate some tension in their abdominal muscles.

During deep inspiration, all the actions of quiet inspiration are increased in extent, but now the auxiliary or accessory muscles provide assistance. It is usual for these accessory muscles to exert tension in a direction opposite to that of their usual or principal function. The deeper and more forced the inspiration, the greater the number of muscles involved, as well as the extent of their activity. The diaphragm, external intercostals, scaleni, and sternocleidomastoids have already been identified. Others can and will play a role. More forceful raising of the ribs can occur using the levatores costarum and serrati posteriores superiores. Tension generated in the sacrospinalis will straighten the vertebral column and raise the ribs even more. Severe air hunger can occur in health with intense anaerobic exercise, or in disease, involving a great many additional muscles, particularly those in the upper respiratory region. Beginning with the alae nasi, which flair the nostrils, and continuing down to include the levator palati, buccinator, platysma, tongue, laryngeal, and posterior neck muscles, all can mobilize to accomplish the task of breathing. Their principal roles are to increase the ease of air inflow by enlarging the air cavities, thus lowering resistance to air movement.

During deep expiration the abdominal wall muscles act significantly to push on the abdominal viscera, as well as flex the vertebral column. Both actions decrease thoracic volume, the former by raising the diaphragm, the latter by lowering the ribs. The internal intercostals also are active, as well as the scaleni. Still others can also play a role, including the quadratus lumborum to fix the lower 2 ribs, and the serrati posteriores inferiores to pull all the other ribs toward these last 2. Thus, there is a considerable reserve of function in the inspiratory muscles other than the diaphragm.

It should also be realized that, during both quiet and deep breathing, the tension generation by inspiratory muscles is not suddenly terminated at the beginning of expiration. There is instead a gradual reduction in tone, and only after the expiration of about 25% of the tidal volume does inspiratory tone finally disappear.

Just as other skeletal muscles can be improved in their performance capacity by both strength and endurance training, so also the respiratory muscles increase their abilities if the training program is of sufficient intensity. These muscles are mosaics of varying cell types, some specialized for strength (the fast-twitch glycolytic-enzyme-emphasizing cells), others for endurance (slow-twitch oxidative-enzyme-emphasizing cells). Primarily strength training, achieved by repeat maximal inspirations and expirations, might yield an increased vital capacity by increasing the functional effectiveness of the glycolytic fibers. Endurance training, such as continued breathing with greater inspiratory resistance, or maintained elevated breathing rates with normal inspiratory resistance, does not appear to change vital capacity, but it does increase the level of maximum sustainable ventilation. This change may occur either through increased enzymatic capabilities of the muscles themselves or through increased neurological mobilization of motor units.

Such training of the breathing musculature is of diverse value. People in competitive sports, where prolonged intense breathing is demanded, until recently have not thought much about the possibility for improved performance through training of their respiratory musculature. Patients of many kinds, particularly with respiratory impairments, such as those caused by cystic fibrosis and chronic obstructive pulmonary disease, can certainly benefit from increased respiratory muscle strength. Patients who are being gradually removed (weaned) from supportive ventilation also need an improvement in strength if they are to successfully re-adapt to normal breathing. An important new thrust in pulmonary medicine is to emphasize evaluation of the muscles of respiration as well as the lungs themselves in total assessment of the function of the entire air pump/gas exchange mechanism.

RELEVANT READING

Anderson, C.L., Shankar, P.S., and Scott, J.H. Physiological significance of sternomastoid muscle contraction in chronic obstructive pulmonary disease. *Respiratory Care* **25**:937–939, 1980.

Belman, M.J., and Sieck, G.C. The ventilatory muscles. Fatigue, endurance and training. *Chest* **82**:761–766, 1982.

Bronk, D.W. and Ferguson, L.K. The nervous control of intercostal respiration. *American Journal of Physiology* **110**:700–707, 1935.

Campbell, E.J.M. *The Respiratory Muscles and the Mechanisms of Breathing.* Year Book Medical Publishers, Chicago, 131 pp. 1958.

Campbell, E.J.M. Physical signs of diffuse airway obstruction and lung distension. *Thorax* **24**:1–3, 1969.

De Troyer, A. Mechanical action of the abdominal muscles. *Bulletin Europeen de Physiopathologie Respiratoire* **19**:575–581, 1983.

De Troyer, A., Kelly, S., and Zin, W.A. Mechanical action of the intercostal muscles on the ribs. *Science* **220**:87–88, 1983.

Loring, S.M. and Mead, J. Abdominal muscle use during quiet breathing and hypernea in uninformed subjects. *Journal of Applied Physiology* **52**:700–704, 1982.

Martin, B.J., Chen, H., and Kolka, M.A. Anaerobic metabolism of the respiratory muscles during exercise. *Medicine and Science in Sports and Exercise* **26**:82–86, 1984.

Pancoast, M.K., Baetjer, F.H., and Dunham, K. Studies on pulmonary tuberculosis. II. The healthy adult chest. *American Review of Tuberculosis* **15**:429–471, 1927.

Raper, A.J., Thompson, W.T. Jr., Shapiro, W., and Patterson, J.L. Scalene and sternomastoid muscle function. *Journal of Applied Physiology* **21**:497–502, 1966.

Roussos, C., and Macklem, P.T. The respiratory muscles. *New England Journal of Medicine* **307**:786–796, 1982.

Shephard, R.J. The maximum sustained voluntary ventilation in exercise. *Clinical Science* **32**:167–176, 1967.

Simpson, L.S. Effect of increased abdominal muscle strength on forced vital capacity and forced expiratory volume. *Physical Therapy* **63**:334–337, 1983.

Taylor, A. The contribution of the intercostal muscles to the effort of respiration in man. *Journal of Physiology* (Lond) **151**:390–402, 1960.

Tenney, S.M. and Reese, R.E. The ability to sustain great breathing efforts. *Respiration Physiology* **5**:187–201, 1968.

Functional Microanatomy of the Respiratory Tract

Chapter Four

Chapter Four Outline

Mechanisms for Modifying the Inspired Air
   A. Mucus and Mucus-producing Cells
   B. Cilia and Cilia-producing Cells
   C. Humidification and Temperature Control

Environmental Effects on Mucosal Function
Defense Against Infection
Location of Specific Cell Types in Respiratory Epithelia

For the lung and its associated passageways to accomplish the task of exchanging large quantities of air between the ambient environment and blood, provision must be made to prevent this exchange from having deleterious effects. The respiratory tract must therefore serve as an effective biologic barrier against air-containing noxious agents and injurious organisms, and must make the gas "palatable" to its surface tissues. It is the purpose of this chapter to briefly outline how the structure of the respiratory tract epithelium accomplishes these ends so well that the tract normally remains sterile from the first bronchial division all the way to the most terminal pulmonary units. We shall learn how the air is warmed, humidified, and cleansed, and how impurities are removed well before the air reaches the bronchial regions of the lung. What happens to the air as it enters the lung itself will be discussed in Chapter Five.

MECHANISMS FOR MODIFYING THE INSPIRED AIR

A. MUCUS AND MUCUS-PRODUCING CELLS

The respiratory tract is lined with an epithelium consisting of ciliated columnar cells, secretory cells, and basal cells all resting on a well-defined basement membrane. Because the basal cells have no contact with the lumen, there is a false appearance of a stratified condition, giving the epithelium its name of *pseudostratified ciliated columnar with mucous cells* (Figure 4-1). This is often simplified as the *respiratory epithelium*. There are additional mucus-secreting structures, the submucosal glands, scattered along the respiratory tract, most notably in the tracheal and bronchial regions. Quantitatively, these produce more mucus than the epithelial mucous cells. The basal cells are the most poorly differentiated of the epithelial cells, and have the potentiality to develop into either ciliated cells or mucous cells.

Lining the respiratory tract is an aqueous mucus secretion, 10 to 20 μm thick. It consists of two layers. The top is a gel layer of hydrated mucus, while underneath lies a less viscous sol layer. The sol layer provides a medium in which cilia can move. The tips of the cilia strike the bottom of the gel layer and propel the mucus toward the mouth. This system must be capable of fine regulation, for even small increases in the dimensions of the aqueous layers lining the trachea and bronchi severely inhibit mucociliary clearance. Similarly, a small decrease in ciliary motion would also have disastrous consequences. The dynamics of regulating the production of mucus from various cells and glands allows just enough, but not an excess, to flow along the respiratory passageway. How this regulation occurs is unknown. Similarly, it is not known how the composition of the mucus lining is regulated to keep just enough sol below the gel portion that the gel does not settle upon the cilia, thereby impeding ciliary actions in mucus motion. It may be that subtle differences in this balance are responsible for the considerable variation of mucus movement. In the trachea, for example, it varies between 7 and 20 mm/min.

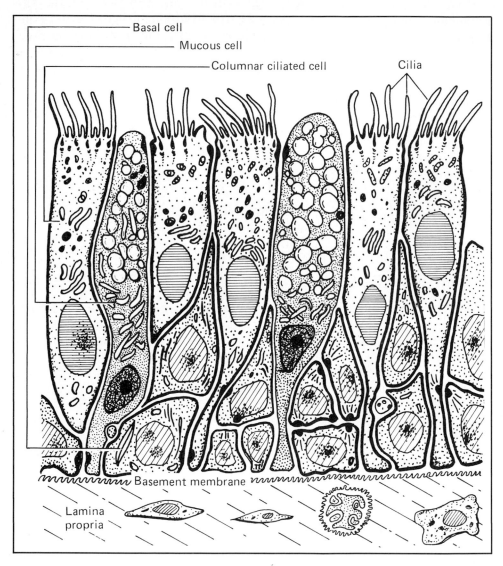

Basal cell

Mucous cell

Columnar ciliated cell

Cilia

Basement membrane

Lamina propria

Figure 4-1.   Sketch of the 'respiratory epithelium' found in much of the upper respiratory tract and as far down as the secondary bronchioles. It is a pseudostratified ciliated columnar epithelium with mucous cells; the various cell types are depicted. [Redrawn with permission from *American Review of Respiratory Disease* 93 (Suppl.) 1–15, 1966.]

Mucociliary transport has long been recognized as an important protective mechanism for clearing inhaled particulate material. Particle sizes greater than or equal to 30 μm deposit in the mouth, larynx, or trachea, whereas particle sizes of 3 μm to 10 μm deposit all along the bronchial tree, as far down as the alveolar ducts. This indicates the effectiveness of mucus as a trap for large quantities of particulate matter. Particle sizes of 1 μm to 3 μm are still able to reach the alveoli. Particles of 0.5 μm or less, while able to access these same regions, are not deposited but simply float around until they are exhaled. For effective mucociliary clearance, the surface of the airways must contain a gel with specific viscoelastic properties. This clearance is determined by the interaction of ciliary activity with the physical properties of the mucus blanket. Recent research has emphasized the mechanisms by which mucus is produced and regulated in its composition such that ciliary activity can effectively control its movement.

Such research studies have not been easy because of several interesting difficulties. First, the mucus secretion is very complex, being produced and modified by a number of mechanisms at several levels within the airways. Second, in the absence of disease, only small amounts of secretion spread out to form a thin layer over the epithelial surface, making it difficult to collect sufficient quantities for study. If sputum is collected and studied, one must contend with the contamination of the respiratory tract portion with salivary secretions. If respiratory secretions are collected from individuals with diseases such as chronic bronchitis, these are not the same as those produced by healthy people. Third, the gel-like secretions are not suitable for standard biochemical analyses.

Analysis of respiratory tract mucus reveals about 95% water and 5% solids. The solids include 2% to 3% proteins and glycoproteins, 1% lipids (mostly phosphatidylcholine), and 1% minerals. The proteins include such familiar substances as albumin, immunoglobins, and fibrinogen, but many other less familiar substances, such as ceruloplasmin (which transports copper), transferrin (which transports iron) and antitrypsin (a bacterial enzyme inhibitor).

The mucus glycoproteins are most responsible for the gelation of airway secretions. A single peptide chain constitutes 10% to 20% of the molecule by weight. The peptide portion has a rather unusual amino acid composition, including about 30% threonine and serine, and 70% proline, glycine, alanine, and hydroxyamino acids. The bulk of the molecule is made up of numerous oligosaccharide chains, 1 to 20 or more sugar residues in length. Several different types of sugar molecules have been identified: fucose, galactose, N-acetylglucosamine, N-acetylgalactosamine, and N-acetylneuraminic acid.

The mucus acts as a viscoelastic gel. When stressed, its response is somewhat intermediate between that of a solid and a liquid. A true solid will be deformed by a stress, but will recover immediately after the stress is removed. A true liquid will also be deformed, and may flow more or less continuously during stress application, but following removal of the stress there will be no recovery to the original shape. Mucus combines both aspects of these extremes of behavior. As described by Malcolm King in 1980, respiratory tract mucus "resembles a well-engineered paint which, when brushed rapidly, flows easily but when the brushing ceases, sticks to the "wall" to which it is applied.

Respiratory tract mucus has essentially two functions. One is to serve as a protective coat against bacteria or inhaled particles. Mucus does not have bacteriostatic action; rather it provides a mechanical barrier to invasion of the bronchial wall by bacteria. The other function is to provide an internal waterproofing action on the wall of the respiratory tract. It covers the tract like a sheet. The meshwork of its long molecules acts like a sponge to hold water, thereby regulating the intake of water by osmosis or the outflow of water by transudation.

Without respiratory tract mucus there would be either shrinkage of the epithelial membranes by desiccation or swelling by edema. Despite the pressure of a barrier to water movement, there is free passage of O_2 and CO_2.

The effect of mucus on water movement can be shown by experiments using eels, which can tolerate osmotic changes when transferred from sea water (hyperosmotic to their body fluids) to fresh water (hypo-osmotic). They can withstand the change because of the protective layer of mucus covering the outside of their body. The mucus can be removed by a solution containing either papain or sodium bicarbonate (1.28 gm/100 ml H_2O). Following this mucus removal, when placed in fresh water they gain weight because of the osmotic inflow of water. They lose weight when immersed in sea water as a result of water efflux from their tissues.

It is difficult to know the exact amount of mucus produced by a healthy person, but estimates have ranged from 10 to 100 ml per day. Disease mechanisms, such as chronic bronchitis, can raise this to as much as 200 ml/day or more. Many airway diseases are characterized by a marked increase in the synthesis of mucus by the bronchial epithelial cells. Those diseases in which this increase is greatest include chronic bronchitis, asthma, infectious pneumonitis and cystic fibrosis. Mucus characteristics may differ among these diseases.

Effective treatment of these disorders may require an ability to control the viscosity, rate of production, and methods of elimination of mucus. To date, research has focused on the physiology of the mucociliary transport system. Further work on the chemistry of respiratory tract mucus is essential to improve the potential for understanding these crucial aspects of the pathogenesis of lung diseases. An important component of respiratory tract mucus are glycoproteins, secreted by epithelial tissues. Some of these secreted mucus glycoproteins have specific antigenic components which are responsible for virus hemagglutination inhibition. Others have components that comprise the blood group substances. The processes which control secretion of the respiratory glycoproteins are largely unknown and are currently a topic of considerable investigation.

A familiar example of a problem with secretions is found in cystic fibrosis, the most common lethal genetic metabolic disease among white children. The incidence of this disease in the United States is about one in 2,000 live births. It is transmitted as an autosomal recessive trait but the defective or absent gene product has yet to be identified. The clinical syndrome associated with cystic fibrosis results in a triad of problems; pancreatic insufficiency (blockage and destruction of pancreatic ducts), elevated sweat electrolytes (particularly sodium and chloride), and chronic pulmonary disease. It is literally a disease of the exocrine glands.

The respiratory tract secretions from people with cystic fibrosis have a 10% to 11% solids content instead of the usual 5% (which could be caused by a shortage of water secretion or an excess of solids production). This relatively large proportion of solids increases the risk of lung infections due to difficulty in maintaining good pulmonary hygiene. The hypoxemia resulting from the impaired gas exchange can result in cor pulmonale (heart disease because of pulmonary complications, e.g., pulmonary hypertension).

Recent studies have indicated that a vigorous exercise program, if begun slowly and done with complete supervision, can help strengthen the respiratory muscles of children with cystic fibrosis, thereby helping them clear their tract of mucus, maintaining better pulmonary hygiene, and improving their lifestyle. Of course, exercise by itself is not enough, but it can supplement the combination of antibiotic therapy, postural drainage, and aerosol treatment that forms the mainstay of care for these patients.

B. CILIA AND CILIA-PRODUCING CELLS

Cilia must be present and functional if mucus is to be kept out of the lungs. They are found in many places in the body: nasal sinuses, eustachian tubes, brain ventricles, oviducts, vasa efferentia, even the inside of the cornea. Typically in the respiratory tract there are about 250 cilia per ciliated cell (Figure 4-2). These are about 6 μm long and 0.2 μm thick. They beat with a rapid propulsive stroke and a slower recovery stroke, about 1,300 times per minute. This means that cilia can move a sheet of mucus about one mm every 3 seconds, or 2 centimeters per minute. A whole new layer of mucus can cover the upper airways every 10 minutes, whereas 30 minutes to an hour is required in the portion below the larynx. The respiratory cilia are bathed in the sol portion of mucus, and their power strokes move the gel portion (Figure 4-3). The recovery stroke occurs just below this height, in the sol portion, allowing no interference with the movement efforts of those cilia contacting the gel layer.

The mystery of how cilia beat has only recently unraveled, with some extremely interesting relationships that led to a better understanding of respiratory physiology. As long ago as 1677, Leeuwenhoek described the swimming movements of spermatozoa, and then much later, in 1834, Purkinje and Valentin described ciliated epithelia. More than 100 years passed until the 1950s when electron microscopists were able to discover that, in both the plant and animal kingdoms, ciliary structure is similar. In addition, all motile cilia have the same basic function, i.e., to move a stream of liquid.

Thus, cilia attached to a moving cell such as a spermatozoon propel it through a liquid, whereas cilia attached to fixed cells, such as those which line the male and female reproductive tracts, or the trachea and bronchial passages, move a liquid over the surface of the cells. The beat pattern is variable. A spermatozoan

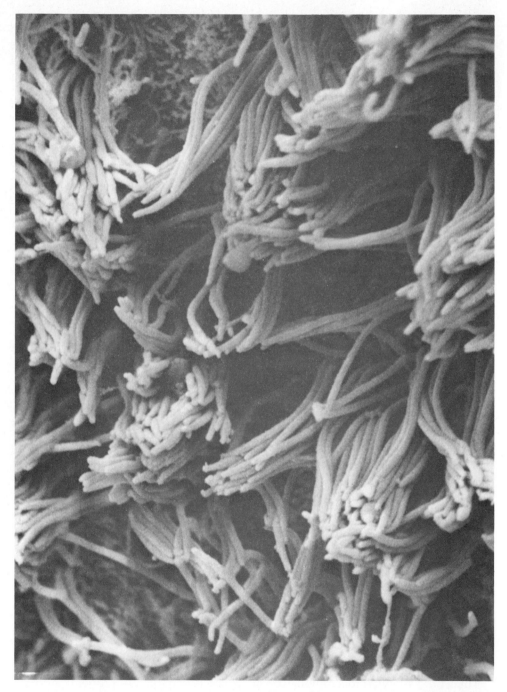

Figure 4-2. Scanning electron micrograph of the ciliated epithelium in the trachea of a rhesus monkey. A few hundred cilia can cover the surface of each cell, serving to propel mucus along the respiratory tract surface. Picture width = 14 μm.

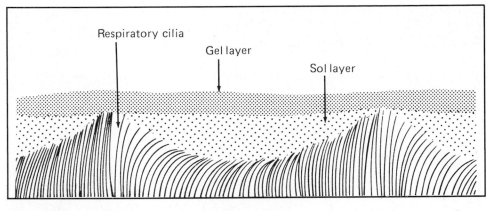

Figure 4-3. Respiratory cilia are bathed in the sol portion of the mucus layer above them. Their power strokes allow mucus movement by contacting the viscous gel layer, always in the same direction.

tail, for example, beats approximately 10 times per second, propagating an undulating wave that moves from the base of the tail to the top to drive the entire cell forward at a rate of from 10 μm to 60 μm per second.

The central core or axoneme of cilia in the respiratory tract is almost identical to a spermatozoan tail. As shown in Figure 4-4a,c there are two central microtubules arranged peripherally to them. Each doublet has an incomplete microtubule attached to a complete microtubule. The doublets are linked together by a filamentous protein called *nexin*. The complete microtubule has two arms of a protein called *dynein*. These point toward the incomplete microtubule of the adjacent doublet (Figure 4-4d).

The dynein arms possess ATP-ase activity, as do radial arms of protein that project from each complete doublet microtubule toward the central pair. The incomplete microtubules have ATP located at various sites along their length, and it is presumed that a similar situation occurs with the central tubules. In the presence of magnesium ions (Mg^{++}), ATP is hydrolyzed and the energy released seems to allow the dynein arms to slide along the incomplete microtubule (Figure 4-4b). This sliding microtubule motion is analagous to the sliding filament hypothesis with actin and myosin in skeletal muscle. A similar attachment, sliding, release and attachment process probably occurs with the radial arms on the central tubules, bending the cilium in a particular direction. The power stroke is ATP-mediated. The dynamics of the recovery stroke, and exactly how it is decided that one side of the cilium will preferentially be the side serving as the power stroke, are still being elucidated. Beat frequency is determined by the amount of ATP present.

This universal mechanism, operant for all types of cilia, explains the etiology of a congenital syndrome resulting from a genetic defect in the synthesis of the protein required for ciliary motion, namely dynein. The immotile cilia syndrome is characterized by a triad of symptoms: sterility in males, chronic sinusitis, and bronchiectasis. In these individuals, their spermatozoa have no motility, and the respiratory tract cilia do not beat. This causes sterility and an increased incidence of respiratory tract infections.

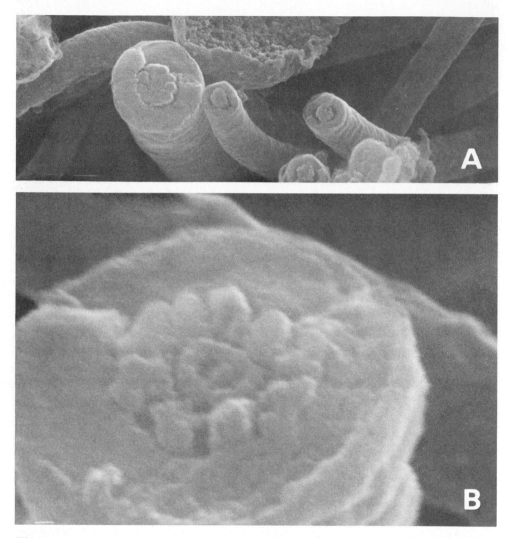

Figure 4-4. Scanning electron micrographs (A, B) of a cilium in cross section, and diagrammed (C, D), showing the outer nine pairs of microtubules and two central microtubules. Each adjacent doublet is interconnected by nexin links, and each connects by spokes to one of the central microtubules. The dynein arms are believed to be involved with ciliary energy transduction in a fashion similar to myosin filaments in muscle, allowing microtubules to move past each other and thereby cause ciliary bending. Figure 4-4 reprinted with permission from Eliasson et al., *New Eng. J. Med.* 297: p. 3, 1977. Picture width of Figures 4-4A and 4B are, respectively, 5 μm and 1 μm.

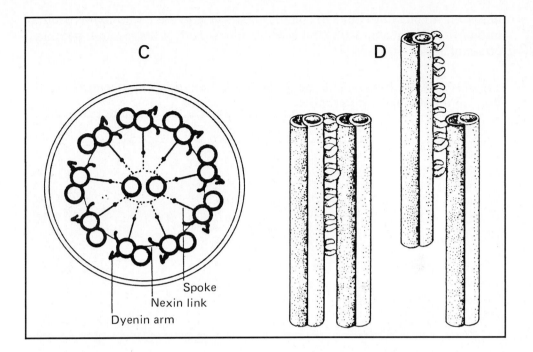

C

D

Spoke
Nexin link
Dyenin arm

C. HUMIDIFICATION AND TEMPERATURE CONTROL

Humidification of the air we breathe usually occurs by water moving from the mucus layer into the inspired air. Thus, very dry air can dehydrate the mucus, increasing its viscosity, thereby slowing or even stopping its flow. This is an important consideration in the design of building air conditioning systems. Excessively dry air can cause discomfort among the building's occupants, with sensations of nasal stuffiness or tracheal congestion.

Exposure of inspired air to the large surface area of the respiratory tract, notably that in the nasal airways, permits virtually complete equilibration to 37° C. This contains 44 mg of water per liter, and exerts a partial pressure of 47 mmHg (6.3 kPa). Thus, the absolute humidity (the amount of water vapor actually present in a given volume of gas) equals the potential water vapor content (the maximum amount of vapor that can be held by a given volume of gas at a particular temperature). The relative humidity in this instance (absolute/potential $\times$ 100) is 100%.

Alveolar air is at body temperature and is saturated with water vapor. Depending on how humid the air is when it is inhaled, more or less water will be added from the mucus to saturate it.

Warm air can contain more water vapor than cold air. Table 4-1 compares the maximum amount of water vapor, along with the accompanying vapor pressure, that can exist in one liter of air at various temperatures. This explains runny noses on a cold day. Cold dry air is inhaled, and then warmed as well as humidified. Upon exhalation the water condenses out at the external nares and accumulates as droplets.

Table 4-1. Curvilinear relationship between increasing temperature and the P_{H_2O} in air at 100% saturation.

Temp, C	P_{H_2O}, mm Hg	P_{H_2O}, kPa
0	4.6	0.61
5	6.5	0.86
10	9.2	1.22
15	12.8	1.70
20	17.5	2.33
25	23.8	3.17
30	31.8	4.23
35	42.1	5.60
37	47.1	6.26
40	55.3	7.35
100	760.0	101.08

The nasal passageways form not only a functional heat exchanger, but also an effective energy conservation mechanism. Air inflow results in humidification and warming, while outflow brings cooling and dehumidification. Usually, inspired air is cooler than body temperature, and the nasal mucosa is cooled somewhat on inspiration. On return to the atmosphere, the expired air warms the mucosa. The vaporization of water upon inspiration requires a considerable energy expenditure, regained during expiration as condensation occurs.

The extent of this mechanism can be better appreciated by imagining a system of breathing with no such return of energy. Arend Bouhuys, in his textbook of respiratory physiology, presented the relevant data for such a system, assuming that an individual inspired air at standard conditions, i.e., completely dry at 0° C. About 2,200 calories per day (9.2 kJ) would be required to evaporate the nearly 420 gm of water to satisfy humidification requirements. This is nearly equal to the entire caloric energy requirement of that individual. Thus, the system we use is enormously advantageous for energy conservation. When air enters the lower portion of the airways by artificial tubing (such as an endotracheal tube), warming and humidification must be supplied mechanically.

The techniques and procedures of aerosol therapy include, along with delivering medications, the humidification of air entering the respiratory passages. Respiratory tract secretions, if they become too viscous from dehydration, increase the risk of infection. Restoration of a normally flowing mucus layer by both the ciliary system and coughing, is greatly enhanced by restoring normal water content in this layer. Nebulizers are devices which will mix water and air in such a way that extremely small water particles of uniform size are produced.

These particles are small enough to penetrate into the farthest reaches of the pulmonary tree where mucus is still found.

ENVIRONMENTAL EFFECTS ON MUCOSAL FUNCTION

The respiratory tract lining is exposed to a wide spectrum of environmental conditions and airborne agents. Many of these agents are small enough to penetrate the farthest reaches of the lungs. It is logical to suspect that the lung should be well equipped with an impressive array of defense mechanisms to keep such agents from entering the body. These mechanisms indeed do exist, but they also have an important responsibility to the lungs, ensuring their ability to serve as effective gas transfer organs.

Being a living tissue, the lung is also subject to modification of its functional state by the environment and by other organs in the body. Several examples can be cited. Dehydration of the epithelium is one important problem. When the ambient humidity is low, the mucus lining cannot provide adequate moisture to humidify effectively the incoming air. The end result is mucosal dehydration, with an increasingly more viscous mucus.

Estrogen hormones tend to increase mucus production as well as its viscosity. Thus, during pregnancy, when circulating blood estrogens increase, it is not unusual to observe mucosal congestion in the respiratory tract.

Anxiety states in many people, as well as states of mild depression, can lead to an excessive secretion of watery mucus. Often there is an associated suspicion of catching a cold because the overt symptoms of a runny congested nose are similar in both. This points out the well-known relationship between positive mental health and good physical health.

Many noxious chemicals exist in the environment which, if inhaled in any quantity, may slow and/or stop ciliary movement. If fresh-air breathing is restored promptly, ciliary motion will resume. However, during the interim, the continuing production of mucus will place an added burden on the cilia, providing a temporary period of mucus congestion. Examples of such irritants include sulfur dioxide, ammonia, and formaldehyde. Man and other species have evolved with a very delicate nasal membrane in relatively direct contact with the environment. They find themselves increasingly challenged as the atmosphere becomes contaminated with the multiple residues of a complex society. Even the gases naturally present—O_2 and CO_2—are not in quantities appropriate for the lungs to directly survive exposure to them. Atmospheric O_2 concentrations are high enough to be marginally toxic, and the CO_2 levels are so low that alkalinization could occur in cells directly exposed. A transportable alveolar environment has evolved to satisfy the dilemmas concerning the crucial gases, separated from the external environment by an appropriately long passageway. But there has been insufficient time to evolve the myriad of mechanisms to cope with technological intrusions into the atmosphere.

Chronic irritation of the respiratory system can have more deleterious effects than acute exposure. The most common form of chronic irritation is by smoke inhaled from cigarettes. The primary problem involves degenerative changes in the respiratory tract epithelium. Associated with this is an increased resultant risk to respiratory infections and the formation of bronchogenic carcinoma.

There are five notable pathological changes occurring from chronic exposure to cigarette smoke. Listed in the sequence that normally develops, these are: 1) depression of ciliary movement, 2) loss of ciliary cells, 3) replacement of such cells by flat squamous cells, 4) increased mucus production by existing goblet cells, and 5) appearance of more goblet cells, thus, more mucus (Figure 4-5). The end result is a chronic bronchitis, complicated by edema of the airways, which produces obstruction to airflow.

One protective mechanism often used to help rid the respiratory tract of this excess mucus secretion is coughing. This explains the increased coughing activity so characteristic of chronic smokers. It is an attempt to cope with the developing chronic obstructive pulmonary disease (COPD). Because COPD in the United States occurs primarily from the effects of cigarette smoking, and because COPD is the second leading cause of worker disability payments, the elimination of such chronic irritation should be useful and desirable for both workers and society.

If the COPD progresses far enough, an increase in macrophage activity in the lung tissue itself, with its accompanying lysosomal destruction of alveolar walls and other connective tissue, diminishes the elastic recoil of the lung. In this condition (emphysema), the elaborate tissue interconnections that ensure small airway patency are compromised, resulting in trapping of air within the lungs and poor ventilation.

The effects of cigarette smoke can affect even those who are adjacent to smokers, but not actually smoking. Young children residing in the homes of smoking parents have a measurably increased incidence of pneumonia and bronchitis during their first year of life. They are sometimes referred to as passive smokers. Similar trends occur in those non-smokers who inhale the smoke of others while working in smoke-filled environments.

The problems associated with marijuana cigarettes are quite different from those with tobacco cigarettes, although marijuana cigarette smokers have a clinically evident increased incidence of bronchitis. First, marijuana cigarettes are never smoked in the quantities indulged in by heavy tobacco cigarette smokers. Second, there is no nicotine in marijuana cigarettes, and thus no attendant cardiovascular risks. Third, the few but very deep inhalations of marijuana smoke permit the various particulate constituents to penetrate the deepest alveoli of the lung. Fourth, with no federal controls over marijuana cigarette composition, particularly with respect to contaminants such as herbicides, in contrast to those with tobacco cigarettes, there is no regulation on the kinds or quantities of such materials that may be included in these cigarettes.

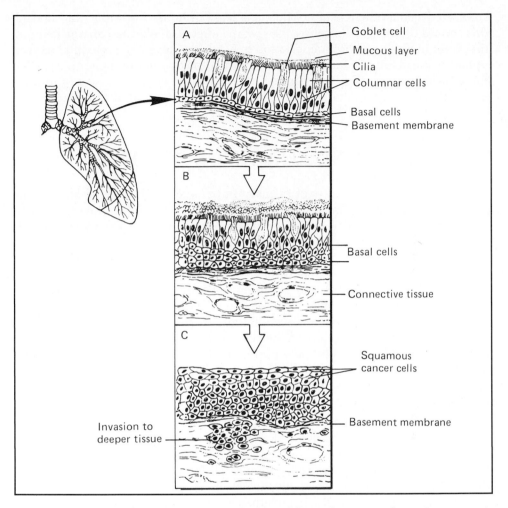

Figure 4-5.   Diagrammatic representation of how the normal respiratory epithelium (A) can be adversely affected through long-term cigarette smoking, first by proliferation of more basal cells, decreased ciliary activity and increased mucus production (B) and later by loss of mucociliary epithelium with replacement by squamous cells that can be the first signs of developing carcinoma. Reprinted with permission from *Principles of Human Anatomy,* by G.J. Tortora, p. 542, Harper & Row, Publishers: New York, 1980.

Fifth, the active psychotropic agent in marijuana cigarettes, i.e., Δ9-tetrahydrocannabinol, is a specific bronchodilator.

This last point emphasizes a problem that must be reckoned with in the performance of aerobic power exercise stress tests. These are work bouts using either a treadmill or bicycle ergometer, with gradually increasing intensity workloads until an individual's maximum or pre-set submaximum performance capacity is achieved. Any subject scheduled to undergo such a test should be counseled against the use of marijuana at least 24 hours prior to it, and if used, this should be noted. Otherwise, the specific effects on elevated airway conduction from the induced bronchodilation may falsely elevate the maximal oxygen uptake value obtained. Temporary discontinuation of other bronchodilators that the subject may be using, which were prescribed clinically, may also be appropriate, depending upon details of their need for onging health maintenance.

DEFENSE AGAINST INFECTION

The mucociliary system is of primary importance in providing an ongoing resistance to infection. Bacteria and viruses will be trapped in the mucus, and moved by cilia, eventually swallowed or expectorated. Viral penetration of cells takes time, and ciliary movement of mucus prevents this. There are an increasing number of soluble chemical factors identifiable in the airway secretions which are important in enhancing defense against infection. Normally, α-1-antitrypsin circulates in blood plasma, and is present on lung surfaces. It can inhibit the activity of bacterial enzymes and lysosomal enzymes, and helps minimize inflammatory reactions that may occur if these enzymes are allowed to act. It may also prevent lung destruction of the type leading to pulmonary emphysema. Lactoferrin is synthesized by polymorphonuclear leukocytes and by glandular mucosal cells. It binds iron, and has a bacteriostatic effect. Lysozyme is a white blood cell enzyme with bacteriostatic properties. It is also on the lower respiratory tract mucosal surface.

The lung is an admirably designed immunologic organ. We have already mentioned its exceedingly rich blood and lymphatic supply, which allows it ample opportunity to circulate not only cells which mediate immunity but also hormonal substances elaborated by other cells. The profoundness of the circulation allows the lung to effectively detect all types of potentially disturbing chemicals and pathogens. By inactivating or removing such noxious agents, the lung serves as an important homeostatic organ.

To the extent that the various immunologic defense mechanisms do not harm the living tissue itself, these processes are of course considered admirable. However, some of these mechanisms are so effective that the lung interstitium may be replaced by fibrotic tissue. Airflow obstruction can also occur by activation of vessel constriction and fluid secretion mechanisms.

It is well known that the immunoglobulins (antibodies present in the serum and external secretions of the body), first isolated in plasma, can be found in the lung. Immunoglobulin A (IgA) is secreted into the respiratory tract, where it has an antitoxin activity, virus neutralization activity, and the ability to activate complement. Complement is a complex system of multiple chemical substances that is an integral part of the body's host defense system.

Immunoglobin E is also found throughout much of the respiratory tract, skin and the cells of mucus membranes, and plays a primary role in prevention of infection. When antigens, such as dust or pollens, enter the lung, they sensitize circulating lymphocytes to differentiate into specialized plasma cells that will release antibodies, including IgE. Asthma is the most well-known example of this so-called immediate hypersensitivity reaction.

Along with plasma cell activation is activation of mast cells which are also found in lung tissue. These cells are at all the key interfaces between the body and external environment (in the skin, lungs, mucosal linings, and in venules). They act as sentinel to invasion by foreign substances. A variety of vasoactive substances (i.e., substances that promote blood vessel constriction or dilation) are produced by these cells, and stored in granules within them. Degranulation of these cells releases the substances into the circulation, mediating what has been called a hypersensitivity reaction. This reaction consists of inflammation (from vasodilation) and bronchoconstriction. Histamine is the substance causing vasodilation. Serotonin is a venoconstrictor. There are several other such substances which will be discussed in Chapter Five. The reactions caused by these substances, e.g., the airway obstruction seen in an asthmatic attack, can be life-threatening, because they are so powerful. In some people, their sensitivity to these agents is excessive.

LOCATION OF SPECIFIC CELL TYPES IN RESPIRATORY EPITHELIA

At the external nares the epithelium is protective in nature, and is stratified squamous non-keratinizing. As one moves into the nasal airways, the classical and so-called respiratory epithelium begins, specialized for warming, cleansing and humidifying. This delicate pseudostratified ciliated columnar epithelium with mucous cells (Figure 4-1) has already been described. It rests upon a continuous basement membrane of varying thickness. Beginning here, and extending all along the respiratory tract, lymphoid aggregates of various sizes and shapes are found in the underlying submucosa. In some instances these accumulations are sizable, such as in the tonsils located in the soft palate region. They are found in all mammals studied, and even appear in animals raised in a germ-free environment. Many of these lymphoid cells contain immunoglobulin A precursors.

Contact of such a delicate surface epithelium with food would not benefit its normal function and could be damaging. Thus, there is an epithelial transition from nasopharynx to oropharynx. Ciliated epithelium with mucous cells gives way to stratified squamous epithelium. Reversion back to the ciliated/mucous cell epithelium will occur at the larynx-trachea intersection (Figure 4-6). In the region of the hard palate, the epithelium has a covering cornified layer composed of hard scale-like cells (Figure 4-7). This layer protects the epithelial cells from damage when solid food is chewed.

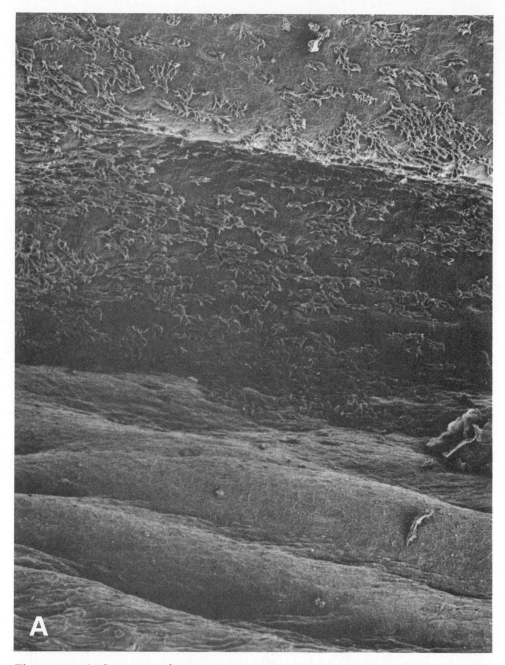

Figure 4-6. A. Scanning electron micrograph of the transition region from pseudostratified ciliated columnar epithelium with mucous cells to stratified squamous epithelium at the junction between nasopharynx (top) and oropharynx (bottom) in the rhesus monkey. Picture width = 385 μm. B. Higher-power view of the oropharynx near the transition, showing more clearly the individual ciliated and squamous cells. Picture width = 87 μm.

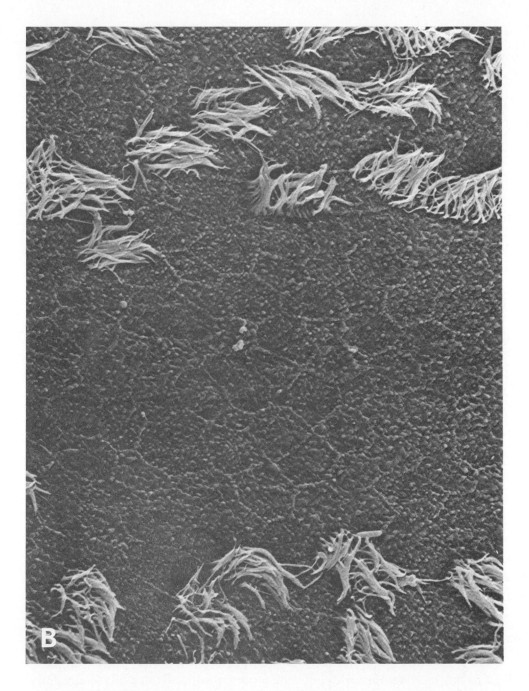

Moving into the laryngeal region, since food and water can still contact the epiglottal portion of the epithelium, one finds that the stratified squamous nonkeratinizing layer still prevails. Just below the epiglottis, through the vocal cord region, the respiratory epithelium is regained. Submucosal mucus-secreting glands are present here, as well as lymphatic tissue.

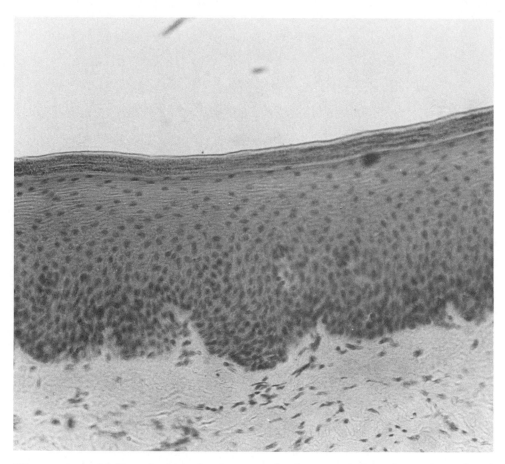

Figure 4-7.   Light micrograph showing the keratinized surface of the hard palate in the human. Stratified squamous epithelium is below it. Picture width = 587 μm.

The lower respiratory tract consists of the trachea, bronchi, and all other respiratory passageways penetrating the innermost portions of the lungs. This is typically divided into a conducting portion, intended to move air from the outside environment to the functional units of the lung and back again, and a respiratory portion, in which gaseous exchange between air and blood occurs. Only the tracheal portion of the lower respiratory tract will be discussed here, with the remainder considered in Chapter Five with lung structure and function.

The respiratory epithelium covers the entire tracheal lumen, even that portion not having cartilaginous rings, i.e., the portion positioned dorsally (posteriorly) and comprised of trachealis muscle. The very high concentration of mucous cells in the trachea, as many as one per 5 ciliated cells—adds to the great mucus-producing capabilities of this region.

The respiratory tract mucosa has a third layer in addition to the epithelial cells and basement membrane. That is the lamina propria *(Figure 4-8)*, which contains

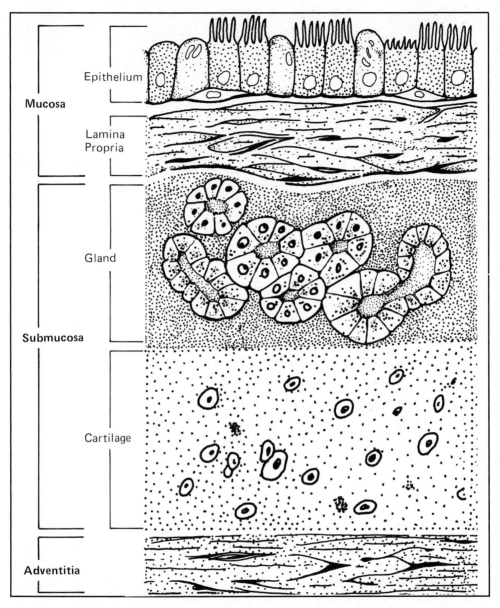

Figure 4-8. Various tissue layers in the trachea, illustrating not only the epithelium but also the underlying lamina propria of the mucosa. Submucosal glands below this, whose ducts reach the tracheal lumen, allow secretory contribution to the mucus layer. Incomplete cartilaginous rings ensure a noncollapsible tube for airflow.

smooth muscle cells, elastic connective tissue fibers, blood vessels, and various cells that can migrate into and out of the bloodstream. Below this is the submucosa, which is considerably more developed in the upper airways and especially in the trachea, where numerous mucus glands have their ducts extending onto the lining surface (Figure 4-8). These glands produce the serous component of tracheal mucus and are capable of discharging considerable volumes of mucus onto the tracheal surface upon stimulation by irritant substances.

A very important cell type found in both the lamina propria and submucosa is the mast cell. This cell is 12 μm to 15 μm in diameter, has a cytoplasm with secretory granules that contain vasoactive substances, and can migrate into the airway lumen, eventually reaching even alveolar spaces. One of its important secretory substances is histamine. Although histamine may produce arteriolar dilation and venoconstriction, it also causes bronchoconstriction. The role of mast cells in the hypersensitivity reaction typified by asthma has already been mentioned.

RELEVANT READING

Afzelius, B. Immotile cilia syndrome and ciliary abnormalities induced by infection and injury. American Review of Respiratory Disease **124**:107–109, 1981.

Boat, T.F., and Cheng, P.W. Biochemistry of airway mucus secretions. Federation Proceedings **39**:3067–3074, 1980.

Bouhuys, A. Breathing. Grune and Stratton, New York, p. 25, 1974.

Eliasson, R., Mossberg, B., Camner, P., and Afzelius, B.A. The immotile cilia syndrome. New England Journal of Medicine **297**:1–6, 1977.

Gail, D.B., and Lenfant, C.J.M. Cells of the lung: Biology and clinical implications. American Review of Respiratory Disease **127**:366–387, 1983.

Hammond, E.C. The effects of cigarette smoking. Scientific American **207** (1): 39–51, 1962.

Hayashi, M. and Huber, G.L. Airway Defenses. Seminars in Respiratory Medicine, **1**:233–239, 1980.

Hinds, W.C. The lung and the environment. Seminars in Respiratory Medicine **1**:197–210, 1980.

Hinds, W.C. and First, M.W. Concentrations of nicotine and tobacco smoke in public places. New England Journal of Medicine **292**:844–845, 1975.

King, M. Viscoelastic properties of airway mucus. Federation Proceedings **39**:3080–3085, 1980.

Lach, E. and Schachter, E.N. Marijuana and exercise testing. New England Journal of Medicine **301**:438, 1979.

Niewoehner, D.E., Kleinerman, J., and Rice, D.B. Pathologic changes in the peripheral airways of young cigarette smokers. New England Journal of Medicine **291**:755–758, 1974.

Phipps, R.J. The airway mucociliary system. *International Review of Physiology* **23:**213–260, 1981.

Reid, L.M., and Jones, R. Mucous membrane of respiratory epithelium. *Environmental Health Perspectives* **35:**113–120, 1980.

Rhodin, J.A.G. Ultrastructure and function of the human tracheal mucosa. *American Review of Respiratory Diseases* **93:**1–15, 1966.

Sturgess, J.M. Structure of the human airway mucosa. *Seminars in Respiratory Medicine* **5:**301–307, 1984.

Tashkin, D.P., Shapiro, B.J., Lee, Y.E., and Harper, C. Subacute effects of heavy marijuana smoking on pulmonary function in healthy man. *New England Journal of Medicine* **294:**125–129, 1976.

White, J.R., and Froeb, H.F. Small-airways dysfunction in nonsmokers chronically exposed to tobacco smoke. *New England Journal of Medicine* **302:**720–723, 1980.

Yarnal, J.R., Golish, J.A., Ahmad, M., and Tomashefski, J.F. The immotile cilia syndrome. *Postgraduate Medicine* **71** (2): 195–217, 1982.

Functional Microanatomy of the Lung

Chapter Five

Chapter Five Outline

Bronchi and Bronchioles
Alveolar Ducts, Alveolar Sacs, and Alveoli
Metabolic Functions of the Lungs
Reactivity of the Airways
  A. Fibrous Framework of the Lungs
  B. Innervation of the Lungs
  C. Alteration of Airway Reactivity by Phamacologic Agents

Of all the major organs in the body, the lung has been one of the most elusive in allowing the accurate description and understanding of its microscopic structure. In most mammals the lungs are the largest organs in terms of volume, but the smallest in terms of relative tissue mass. The incredible complexity of the airways, as well as the problems of preparing and viewing such delicate tissue have been formidable. It was only as late as 1952 when F.N. Low and C.W. Daniels used electron microscopy to conclude that the alveoli really do have a continuous epithelial surface, contrary to the views of many before that time. In 1963 Ewald Weibel described the stereology of the lung; his concept of quantifying the many generations of passageways allowed order out of the chaos that had reigned previously when one attempted to trace the route of air from a large bronchus to a small alveolus. A few years later, in 1967, W.M. Thurlbeck, using light microscopy, emerged with the now-familiar values of about 60 square meters (m^2) for the alveolar surface area of a lung containing 5 liters of air, and about 48 m^2 for the capillary surface area. It remained for Weibel to learn by electron microscopy studies that those values are in fact much larger (more like 160 and 158 m^2, respectively, because of extensive surface corrugations). Current anatomical studies have been focusing more specifically on the cellular ultrastructure and function in the lung. The lung cells have become far more than a structural framework for tubes allowing airflow. The secretion of substances, such as surfactant, an elaborate immunological defense mechanism, and an important role in metabolizing substances produced elsewhere has led to consideration of the lung as a mosaic of diverse function, more interesting to study as more is learned.

BRONCHI AND BRONCHIOLES

The anatomist John Franklin Huber first elucidated what he termed as "the fundamental concept" in understanding lung structure and function. As he wrote in 1949, "very simply stated, this concept is that the lung in its ultimate analysis is the complete or total branching of the bronchus leading to the lung." It was Huber who suggested a working terminology for the various bronchopulmonary segments (described in Chapter Two) that is used routinely today. This conceptualization has added enormously to the clinical interpretation of regional lung disorders.

The bronchi and most of the bronchioles comprise the so-called conducting zone of the lung because here no exchange of respiratory gases occurs across their walls. They exist to transport gas from the trachea to the zone where gas exchange does occur. This conducting zone occupies only about 115 cc of the total volume of 5000 cc for the two lungs. The trachea initially divides into two *primary bronchi. Secondary or lobar bronchi* enter each lobe of the lung. Thus, there are three right secondary bronchi (superior, middle, inferior), and two left secondary bronchi (superior, inferior).

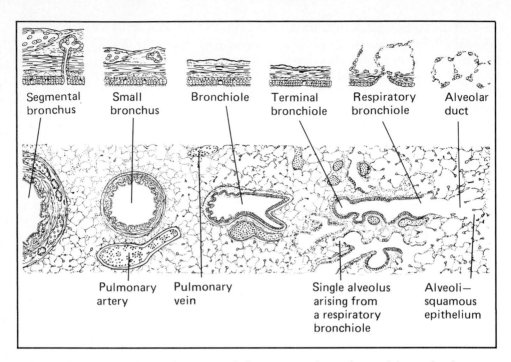

| Segmental bronchus | Small bronchus | Bronchiole | Terminal bronchiole | Respiratory bronchiole | Alveolar duct |

| Pulmonary artery | Pulmonary vein | | Single alveolus arising from a respiratory bronchiole | Alveoli— squamous epithelium |

Figure 5–1.   Histologic features of the various bronchi and bronchioles. Reprinted with permission from *An Atlas of Histology,* by W. H. Freeman and B. Bracegirdle, p. 101 Heinemann Educational Books, Ltd: London, 1966.

These secondary bronchi divide into *tertiary or segmental bronchi* which supply the various bronchopulmonary segments (Chapter Two, *Figure 2-9*) with air. There are 10 right bronchopulmonary segments, and 10 right segmental bronchi. Similarly, there are nine left bronchopulmonary segments, hence nine left segmental bronchi. The segmental bronchi divide further into terminal or subsegmental bronchi (*Figure 5-1*, Table 5-1). These tubes also have cartilage. In fact, the presence of cartilage is an important histologic criterion for considering one of these respiratory passageways as a bronchus rather than a bronchiole.

The larger bronchi will be accompanied by both an artery and a vein, and the cartilaginous tissue rings are very prominent. When one examines horizontal sections through a portion of lung containing bronchi, one can see the lung tissue surrounding them. Easily visible are the various bronchial branches. This lung substance is sometimes also termed pulmonary interstitium or parenchyma. It is a supporting reticular network of connective tissue into which the various lung airways and blood vessels are arranged.

Pseudostratified ciliated columnar epithelium with mucous cells—the familiar respiratory epithelium—lines all of the bronchi. There are a large variety of epithelial cell types in this bronchial epithelium whose importance is just beginning to be elucidated. We have already described the ciliated cells, mucous (goblet) cells, and basal cells, present in the nasal cavities, nasopharynx, and

TABLE 5-1.   Subdivisions of the Respiratory Tree

Generation	Name	Diameter cm	Length cm	Number per Generation	Histological Notes
0	Trachea	1.8	12	1	Wealth of mucous cells
1	Primary Bronchi	1.2	4.8	2	Right larger than left
2	Lobar Bronchi	0.8	0.9	5	3 right, 2 left
3	Segmental Bronchi	0.6	0.8	19	10 right; 8 left
4	Subsegmental Bronchi	0.5	1.3	20	
5 ↓ 10	Small Bronchi	0.4 0.1	1.1 0.5	40 1,020	Still have cartilage; many cell types as well as respiratory epithelium
11 ↓ 13	Bronchioles: Primary & Secondary	0.1 0.1	0.4 0.3	2,050 8,190	No cartilage; smooth muscle, cilia, mucous cells present
14 ↓ 16	Terminal Bronchioles	0.1 0.1	0.2 0.2	16,380 32,770	No mucous cells; smooth muscle, cilia, and cuboidal cells
16 ↓ 20	Respiratory Bronchioles	0.1 0.1	0.2 0.1	65,540 262,140	No smooth muscle; cilia, cuboidal cells; cilia disappear
21 ↓ 23	Alveolar Ducts	0.05 0.04	0.1 0.05	524,290 8,390,000	No cilia; cuboidal cells
24	Alveoli+	244	238	300,000,000	

*Adapted from E. R. Weibel, *Morphometry of the Human Lung*, Springer Verlag: Berlin, 1973.
+Alveolar dimensions given in micrometers.

trachea as well. Other specialized cells exist. *Clara cells* are present and numerous, especially in small bronchi and bronchioles. They are secretory, but the secretion is not known. Some have suggested that they secrete the sol portion of the mucus lining. Others have implicated a role for them in producing a surface-tension-lowering agent for the non-alveolar regions which have no cartilaginous support, such as the distal bronchioles. The patency of these small bronchioles could probably never be regained if they collapsed at very low lung volumes. The secreted material is not surfactant, however. They can differentiate into ciliated cells when subjected to irritants. *Serous cells* are most prevalent in the trachea, but everywhere they are located they produce a fluid that becomes part of the total airway mucus secretion. The serous fluid, however, is less viscous than the mucous cell secretion. *Brush cells* are found here, as elsewhere in the airways.

Their microvilli suggest some kind of absorptive function. *Kultschitzsky cells* (sometimes called argyrophilic cells because their cytoplasmic granules avidly take up silver stains when prepared for study using transmission electron microscopy) are very common in the fetal and neonatal stages of development, but are rare in adults. They appear to secrete pharmacologically active substances (called amines because they contain amino (NH_2) groups). Their functional significance remains unclear.

The entire bronchial mucosa is provided with *epithelial tight junctions* which form from fusion of adjacent epithelial cell membranes. This very effectively prevents any materials, wanted or unwanted, from being deposited in the bronchial tissue itself. It is one of the body's least permeable epithelial layers. The presence of small nerve endings just below these tight junctions, in the intercellular space, suggests a mechanism for the bronchoconstriction and rapid shallow breathing that can occur when inhaled noxious substances, such as ozone, reach this part of the lower respiratory tract. They may be the afferent limb of this "irritant reflex." If adversely affected by such substances, the permeability of these tight junctions could reduce the effectiveness of the bronchial mucosa as a barrier to the outside world. Subsequent exposure to such noxious agents could result in a more pronounced constrictor response.

In addition to the epithelium, there are submucosal glands, which can increase their structural complexity markedly with chronic stimulation by noxious substances, such as cigarette smoke. This occurs in chronic bronchitis, which is a common sequel to long-term cigarette smoking. In fact, hypertrophy of the submucosal glands seems to correlate rather well with habits that include excessive cigarette smoking. Bronchial glands are under parasympathetic nervous system (cholinergic) control, and when stimulated they empty their contents into the bronchial lumen. Some secrete predominantly a serous fluid, others preferentially secrete mucus.

Particles less than 3 μm in diameter remain suspended in bronchial air and pass into bronchioles, where, if they are greater than 1 μm, they will be trapped in bronchiolar mucus. Particles greater than 3 μm in diameter never move farther than the bronchi. Particles smaller than 1 μm may reach the alveoli and will be picked up by alveolar macrophages.

Bronchioles have a diameter of less than 1 mm, and no cartilaginous supporting elements. There is only an accompanying pulmonary arteriole, not a venule. They have the largest amount of smooth muscle in their walls relative to their diameter, with fibers arranged both circularly and longitudinally. Hence, contraction of this smooth muscle can greatly vary both bronchiolar airway diameter and length. The largest of these airways are the primary and secondary bronchioles *(Figure 5-2a)*. They have plenty of smooth muscle, as well as cilia and mucous cells—the typical respiratory epithelium, although mucous cells are considerably fewer in number compared to the trachea and bronchi *(Figure 5-2b)*.

It is in the bronchiolar region of the lung that some of the greatest manifestations of disease are evident. Bronchospasm obstructs the bronchi. The bron-

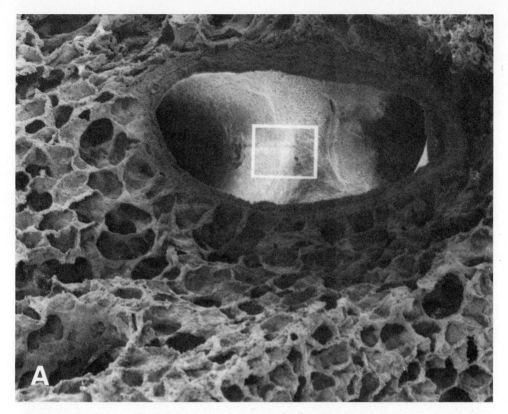

Figure 5-2 A.   Scanning electron micrograph of rhesus monkey primary bronchiole, showing its bifurcation into two daughter airways. The thick connective
tissue wall is in contrast to the very thin walls of surrounding alveoli. (Picture
width: 1 cm = 74 μ).

chioles can also be involved. Air becomes trapped within these bronchioles. The
tighter the trap closes, the harder it is to breathe, and a fear of suffocation can
develop. In asthmatic attacks the secretion of mucus, which is difficult to expel
and often present in large amounts, not only occludes the lumen of the bronchi
and bronchioles, but also traps inspired air in the alveoli. In asthma, mucus
glands are larger and more numerous than normal. Unfortunately, the ciliated
epithelium necessary for mucus transport may be eroded or replaced by more
mucus-producing mucous cells.

Following the secondary bronchioles, *terminal bronchioles* appear *(Figure 5-3
A, B).* These have smooth muscle and ciliated cuboidal cells, but no mucous
cells. Alveoli may be attached to them along their sides, but the walls are too
thick with elastic connective tissue to allow diffusion of gases across them. It is
in fact the elastic aspects of these walls that are largely responsible for maintaining their patency.

There is a *transition zone* in the lung, consisting of the final bronchiolar divi-

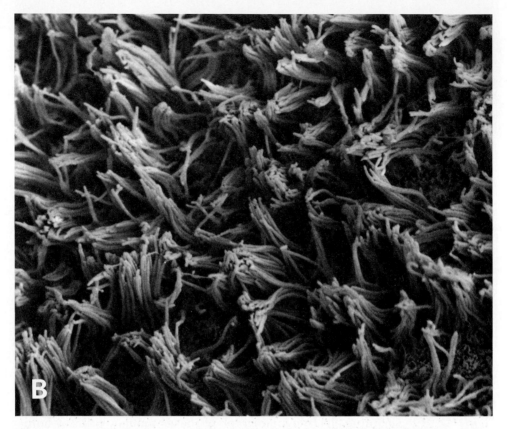

Figure 5-2 B.   Enlargement of a portion of the bronchiolar epithelium within the box in Figure 2-A reveals a preponderance of ciliated cells, with mucous-producing goblet cells (mc) identifiable by the brush microvilli on their surface. (Picture width: 1 cm = 1.7 μ).

sion, the *respiratory bronchioles*. These have no smooth muscle—just squamous and cuboidal cells, and ciliated cells in the upper portions. Alveolar outpocketing can occur, thus, a small amount of respiratory gas exchanges with the bloodstream. It is in this transitional zone that the mixing area for alveolar gas, inspired gas, and dead space gas resides. There are a few generations of these bronchioles and the more distal ones have more alveoli. These are part of a long-defined but poorly understood unit called the lung *acinus*. As long ago as 1872, Rindfleisch coined this term to refer to what he envisioned as the functional pulmonary unit. It included what is beyond a terminal bronchiole, i.e., respiratory bronchioles, alveolar ducts and alveoli. Presently it is estimated that each lung has about 150,000 such structures.

The respiratory bronchioles occupy about 875 cc of total lung volume. With conducting tissue occupying another 125 cc of volume, this means that about 3,000 cc will comprise the respiratory zone. The remaining 1,000 cc of lung volume is occupied by blood vessels, connective tissue, and other tissues.

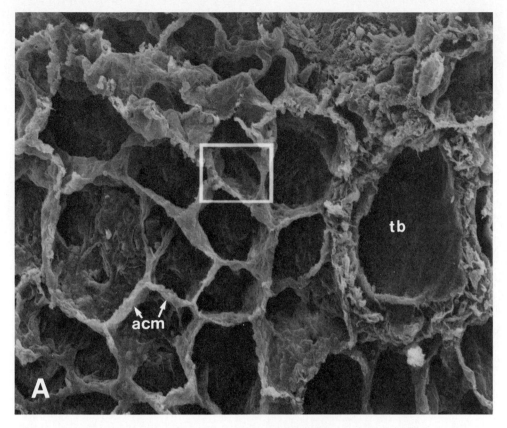

Figure 5-3 A.   Scanning electron micrograph of rhesus monkey terminal bron-chiole (tb), surrounded by alveoli. The alveolocapillary membranes (acm) are much thinner than the bronchiolar membrane, permitting rapid gas transfer between alveolus and capillary. Compare the wall of this terminal bronchiole with the much thicker primary bronchiole in *Figure 5-2 A*. (Picture width: 1 cm = 33.5 μ).

ALVEOLAR DUCTS, ALVEOLAR SACS, AND ALVEOLI

An *alveolar duct* resembles a long corridor with rooms adjacent to each other on the sides; the rooms are *alveoli (Figure 5-1)*. Each duct ends in an *alveolar sac*. The alveoli are about 240 μm in diameter, and number about 300 million in the 2 lungs. Functionally, this is where most gas exchange occurs. A typical distance from the cricoid cartilage to an alveolus might be about 24 cm, although consid-erable variation exists. However, at least 12 cm is accounted for by the trachea alone. Only in the final 7 of the 24 generations of branching (i.e., respiratory bronchioles and beyond), does gaseous exchange occur. The movement of air in these regions is achieved by diffusion; pressure-oriented flow appears to be

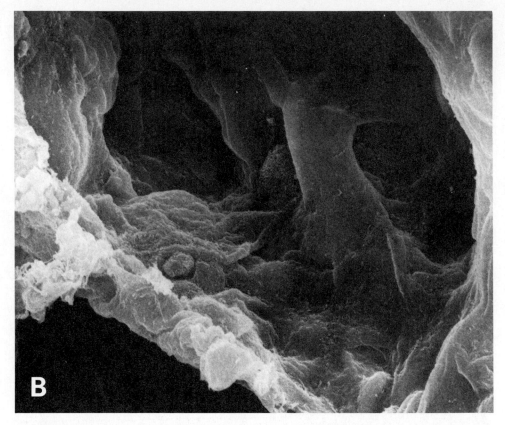

Figure 5-3 B.   Enlargement of part of the area within the box in *Figure 3-A* shows detail of the alveolar surface. This is comprised chiefly of membranous pneumonocytes (Type I cells). (Picture width: 1 cm = 3.46 μ).

lacking. This is, of course, a legacy of the enormous increase in total cross-sectional area after the 18th generation. Notice in Table 5-1 the increase in cross-sectional area that must occur between the final few generations as the number of each unit subdivision increases.

In addition to this airflow route, there is some mixing of alveolar air between adjacent alveoli through inter-alveolar *pores of Kohn*. Although only 5 μm to 10 μm wide, these are well-accepted as one means for collateral ventilation of air within acini. They also have the possibility of equalizing pressure gradients among alveoli, and serve as an intra-alveolar route of transit for wandering alveolar macrophages. Another collateral connection is the accessory bron-chioalveolar *canals of Lambert*, which are as much as 30 μm in diameter. These allow principally intraacinar collateral ventilation.

A variety of specific cell types exist in the alveolar region of the lung, some forming the alveolar epithelium. *Alveolar Type I* cells comprise about 40% of the total number of alveolar epithelial cells, but 93% of the alveolar surface. Because

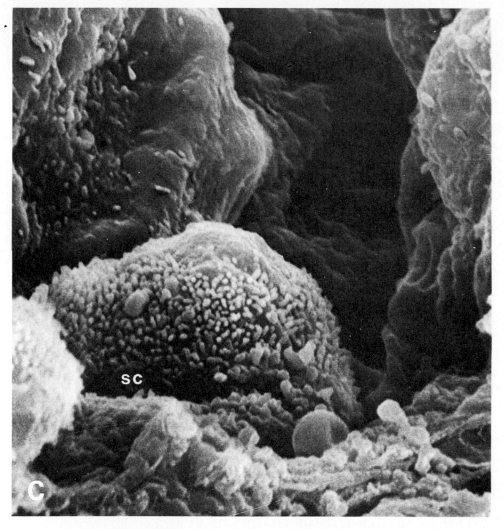

Figure 5-3 C.   The surfactant-producing (Type II) cells (sc) are identified easily by the presence of brush microvilli on all except the bald top of their round luminal surface. (Picture width: 1 cm = 0.85 µ).

of their extremely attenuated cytoplasm, in some regions they are almost invisible using light microscopy. It is this thinness, coupled with very little intracellular organelle development, that maintained the controversy for such a long time over the existence of a continuous epithelial lining. It has now become clear that these cells have their cytoplasm so attenuated that they actually extend into as many as half a dozen adjacent alveoli, forming part of their walls as well. These cells do not seem to undergo mitotic division; there would be considerable disruption of alveolar integrity if such occurred.

Alveolar Type II cells have been studied in great detail because it was discovered in 1954 that they produce pulmonary surfactant. This alveolar lining layer has important surface-tension-lowering characteristics which will be described in detail in Chapter Seven. They are relatively small in size compared to Type I cells, but occur in considerably greater numbers. They are easily identified using scanning electron microscopy, by the presence of brush microvilli on their surface *(Figure 5-3C)*. Inside these cells are all the specializations required for mass production of their secretion: plenty of stored lipids and phospholipids, mitochondria, Golgi apparatus, and endoplasmic reticulum. In addition to secretion, they are also the primary stem cells in the alveolar epithelium, being able to rapidly multiply in numbers when oxidative or other injurious agents penetrate this region. They can also differentiate into Type I cells.

Since pulmonary capillaries course along the alveoli, they obviously come into intimate contact with both Type I and Type II cells. Thus, the so-called air-blood barrier can conceivably be only two cell layers thick (plus two basement membranes) *(Figure 5-4)*. This barrier typically is about 1.0 μm thick, although a small amount of interstitial tissue often thickens it somewhat. Not only do gases diffuse easily across this barrier, but also Type I cells actively phagocytose intra-alveolar particles, as well as proteins, releasing them into the interstitial space or into the plasma. This is one of the mechanisms for clearing the lungs of fluid following aspiration of fresh water during a near-drowning episode, and just following birth.

The *alveolar macrophage* has the job of keeping the alveoli clean and sterile. Particles smaller than 2 μm can access the alveoli, and they are ingested by these macrophages, about 15 μm to 30 μm in diameter. When active, the cells have plenty of mitochondria and hydrolytic-enzyme-containing lysosomes for maintaining a rapid rate of processing the ingested debris. They are bactericidal and ingest these disease agents. Increases or decreases in the numbers of circulating lung macrophages are directly related to an individual's resistance to lung infections. Attenuation of macrophage activity can occur with the presence of cigarette smoke, hypoxia, hyperoxia, ozone, nitrogen dioxide, ethanol ingestion, and corticosteroid ingestion.

The alveolar macrophage derives from the bone marrow, and is a specialized form of monocyte, surviving as long as 2 months in the lung. It moves into the respiratory tract by mechanisms little understood at present, giving up a protected life of being bathed by blood for the stresses of a high O_2 environment with direct exposure to air, toxins, and microbes. Phagocytosis is an energy-dependent process, and these cells have the highest metabolic rate of any mammalian phagocytic cell. Not only is there an elevated O_2 production, but also an increase in hydrogen peroxide, which is destroyed by the enzyme catalase. Macrophages actively wander from one alveolus to another, crossing via pores of Kohn. They can divide while residing in the lung. This helps maintain their numbers. Others are decimated constantly as they move up the respiratory tract by their own and ciliary movement, only to be swallowed, destined for digestion in the stomach. The macrophage cell membrane is specialized for recognition of foreign materials by the presence of receptors for Immunoglobulin G and for certain components of the complement cascade. Very often antigenic particles become op-sonized, i.e., coated with serum that contains immunoglobulins and complement. Opsonization renders the alveolar macrophages more functional at antigen detection, and the antigens more vulnerable to phagocytosis.

METABOLIC FUNCTIONS OF THE LUNGS

Until recently, functions of the lung other than those related to gas exchange between the capillary blood and the atmosphere have generally been ignored. This is caused by the technical difficulties encountered in *in vivo* measurements of metabolic gas exchange of an organ whose principal function is to exchange the same gases between the atmosphere and the blood in the pulmonary capillary bed. However, it has long been apparent that the lungs were the only organ of the body through which all the circulating blood volume passes. It is not surprising, therefore, that as investigative techniques have improved, the lung has been found to have a multitude of functions other than gas exchange. These functions can affect the physiology of every organ in the body. The challenge has been to mix anatomy with physiology and to identify from a cellular viewpoint how each function is performed.

Clearly, disease involving the lungs must have significant effects on these non-gas-exchanging functions of the lung, which will become increasingly important in understanding the multi-system disease patterns. In addition, prolonged partial cardiopulmonary bypass is coming into vogue as a form of therapy for several forms of pulmonary failure and/or cardiogenic shock. This technique provides only the gas exchanging functions of the lungs. It remains to be seen what will be the effects of prolonged cardiopulmonary bypass on the interacting organ systems of the body.

Probably the best studied metabolic activity of the lungs is the biosynthesis of *surfactant,* whose principal ingredient is a phospholipid commonly called lecithin (actually dipalmitoylphosphatidylcholine or DPPC). This molecule contains fatty acids and choline esterified to the glycerol moiety of triglyceride. The fatty acids required for the synthesis of DPPC and other phospholipids in surfactant are either derived from the circulating free fatty acids or are obtained by the action of pulmonary lipases on triglycerides extracted from the circulation. In addition, the lungs can synthesize fatty acids from glucose. Regardless of the form of fatty acid acquisition, the synthesis of DPPC requires energy derived from glucose metabolism. These surface-active phospholipids are stored within the lamellar bodies of the granular pneumonocytes. The importance of this material in stabilization of the lungs will be discussed in Chapter Seven.

Another major metabolic activity includes the role of lung tissue on *vasoactive substances*—molecules with specific actions on the smooth muscle of arterioles and bronchioles. In the lung there is both synthesis and breakdown of such substances, with both constriction and dilation possible. Bronchoconstriction and bronchodilation, vasoconstriction and vasodilation, and capillary permeability changes are all physiological responses with important consequences for lung function in diffuse lung injury. The clear establishment of cause and effect relationships has been difficult. Not only can microvascular injury cause a complicated series of events which release some of these substances, but also the existence of such substances in the blood from antigenic and other reasons can also produce vascular and airway response changes. During the 1970s and 1980s this topic has been one of enormous research interest, with breakthroughs in many significant areas.

One important area involves an increased understanding of the role of endothelial cell surfaces. We now know that capillaries and arterioles are not merely tubes through which blood flows. Rather, the presence of enzymes and receptors on the endothelial cell surfaces permits the synthesis or breakdown of many substances which in turn affect vessel patency. The vast size of the pulmonary blood vessel network, as well as the delicate fluid balance that must remain between the lung interstitium and blood vessels to prevent pulmonary edema, suggest physiologic regulation of profound importance for health and disease.

There is no other vascular bed in the body which comes in contact with the entire cardiac output. As such, then, it is by far the largest vascular bed, its size staggering the imagination. J.W. Ryan and U.S. Ryan have suggested that it may have 1,500 miles of vessels, with as little as one milliliter of blood able to be spread out over 70 miles of capillaries. With about 70 ml of blood in the pulmonary capillaries at any moment in the average resting adult, most of the bed is relatively nonperfused. But during exercise the possibilities for accommodating increased flow requirements are enormous.

Another important topic relates to an improved understanding of the function of mast cells described in Chapter Four. The existence of these cells in the lungs, with their roles in reacting to antigenic substances by release of vasoactive agents, makes the lung a prime target for the full manifestation of their effect. Thus, an understanding of bronchiolar and lung vascular responses to diseases involves an interactive understanding of mast cell and endothelial cell physiology. Several examples of the interaction of vasoactive substances with the lung were mentioned in Chapter Four. Mast cells, for example, produce serotonin, a venoconstrictor and bronchoconstrictor, and histamine, a vasodilator. Inactivation of serotonin occurs in the lungs, but histamine is unaffected.

Bradykinin and angiotensin II are two other vasoactive agents that can be, respectively, inactivated and activated by the action of dipeptidyl carboxypeptidase, an enzyme on the luminal surface of pulmonary endothelial cells. Bradykinin is a vasodilator normally produced by the action of any of a group of proteolytic enzymes called kallikreins. Angiotensin is a substance with functions relating both to electrolyte balance and vasoconstriction. It is produced initially in an inactive form (angiotensin I) in response to a lowered renal blood pressure. Juxtaglomerular cells in the kidney, sensitive to blood pressure changes, increase the release of their enzyme renin *(Figure 5-5)*. In turn, renin cleaves angiotensin I, containing 10 amino acids, from a much larger and nor-

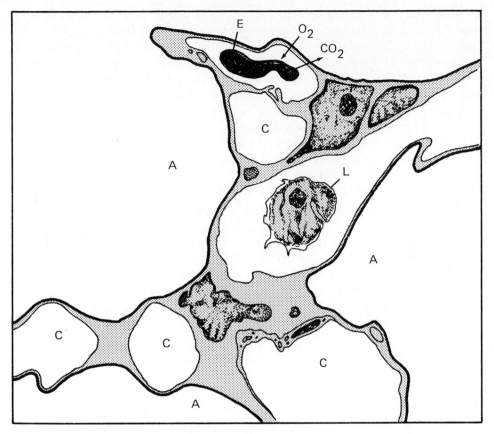

Figure 5-4. Sketch of the alveolocapillary membrane, showing relationships between the basement membranes of alveolus (A) and capillary, type I structural cells in the alveolar wall (which predominate in terms of surface area), type II surfactant-producing cells also in the alveolar wall, and the narrow capillary lumen, which typically is barely large enough for erythrocytes to move through without distortion. Sketch shows pulmonary capillary (C) with erthyrocyte (E), and another capillary containing a lymphocyte (L)

mally circulating plasma protein called angiotensinogen. This decapeptide is then converted to an octapeptide, angiotensin II, by cleavage of two more amino acids, as it passes lung endothelial cells. Whereas angiotensin I has no biologic activity, angiotensin II is an extremely potent vasoconstrictor.

Logically, one would not prefer angiotensin II to be fully active in the pulmonary arterial circulation—its greatest value is in the systemic arteriolar circulation. Conveniently, as mentioned above, it is produced downstream from the pulmonary arterioles. With a halflife of about 3 minutes, its effects on the pulmonary circulation by the time it returns from the systemic circulation will be minimal.

Arachidonic acid plays a crucial role as the precursor substance for a far-reaching array of substances that affect blood vessel patency, vascular permeability, and accumulation of leukocytes or platelets at sites of vessel injury. Arachidonic acid is a polyunsaturated fatty acid present in cell membranes. Degranulation of mast cells or the activation of phospholipase enzymes by inflammatory stimuli that affect endothelial cells cause liberation of free arachidonic acid. Its metabolism can follow several routes, producing some of the most potent agents known in affecting pulmonary circulation and the extent of diffuse lung injury. Currently, this is an extremely active research area in pulmonary physiology and biochemistry. As further information emerges, a better understanding of cell functions that influence pulmonary system operation should be obtained.

One route is conversion through action of the enzyme lipoxygenase to a series of 20-carbon fatty acid derivatives called leukotrienes (Figure 5-6). Leukotriene D_4 is the most potent and it produces bronchoconstriction. Asthmatic patients are as much as 300 times more sensitive to these substances than unaffected subjects. Leukotrienes may also mediate changes in mucus production, vascular permeability, and mucociliary clearance, all of which are important aspects of human asthma. Leukotrienes C_4, D_4, and E_4 can all increase pulmonary arterial pressure and pulmonary vascular resistance because of their potent actions as pulmonary and systemic vasoconstrictors.

Another route is conversion through the enzyme cyclooxygenase to a group of well-known 20-carbon substances—prostaglandins of the "2" series. (In prostaglandin biochemistry, three series of substances are recognized, depending on whether there are 1, 2, or 3 double bonds at specific carbon atom sites.) As seen in Figure 5-6, from prostaglandin G_2, further syntheses in either endothelial cells or platelets produce other prostaglandins with specific functions. Prostacyclin (PGI_2) inhibits platelet aggregation, and helps maintain the antithrombotic potential of the circulation. It also inhibits platelet serotonin release, and is a vasodilator, helping to ensure blood flow during lung vascular injury. Finally, because it increases the microvascular surface area available for fluid filtration, it increases pulmonary lymphatic flow.

Acting in a fashion almost opposite to prostacyclin is thromboxane A2. This substance is a pulmonary vasoconstrictor, and induces platelet aggregation and neutrophil adherence, all of which contribute to the development of pulmonary edema.

Prostaglandins D_2 and $F_2\alpha$ are potent bronchoconstrictor agents in asthmatic patients, with D_2 being the predominant prostaglandin released from activated human lung mast cells. The interactive effects of these substances with each of the others mentioned above will interest researchers and clinicians for years to come, and the information obtained will be of almost certain improved benefit to the understanding and treatment of the many pulmonary complications of asthma and edema. Acetylsalicylic acid (aspirin), for example, blocks the cyclooxygenase enzyme, and glucocorticoids inhibit the release of arachidonic acid from cell membranes with tissue injury. Further study of these and other drugs will not only enhance knowledge of the physiological mechanisms at

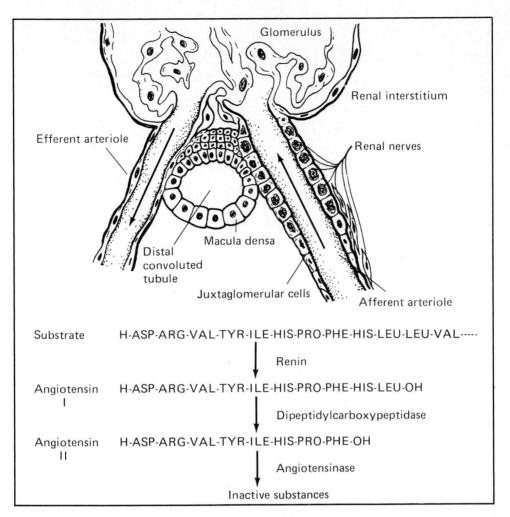

Figure 5-5. Sketch of the juxtaglomerular apparatus in the kidney, site of release of stored renin upon stimulation by situations of low filtration pressure. Renin initiates formation of active angiotensin (II) by cleaving a decapeptide (angiotensin I) from a circulating protein substrate, which subsequently is reduced to the active octapeptide, angiotensin II, by a dipeptidylcarboxypeptidase ('converting enzyme') found primarily in lung tissue. Sketch reprinted with permission from *American Journal of Medicine* 55: 334, 1973.

work, but will allow pharmacologic manipulation of those mechanisms that will benefit patients suffering from situations where the physiological mechanisms have been disrupted.

A topic of considerable recent interest involves the explanation for a complicated combination of clinical symptoms that result following massive lung injury. The syndrome was first described in 1967 as adult respiratory distress

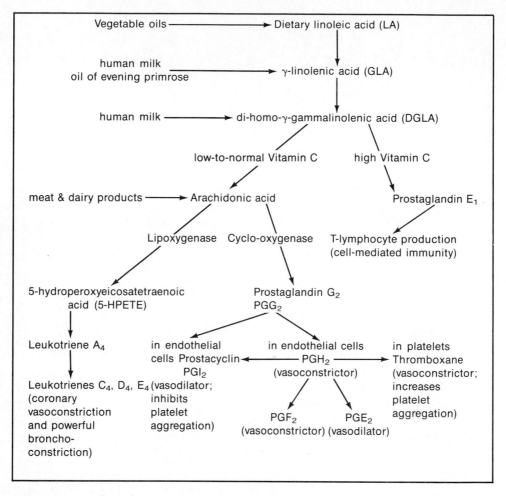

Figure 5-6. Flow diagram integrating current concepts concerning aspects of arachidonic acid production, with its subsequent possible conversion into a whole host of substances having potent activity on smooth muscle that affects bronchiolar as well as arteriolar caliber. Arachidonic acid is an integral part of the structure of cell membranes, released into the circulation when the membrane integrity is disturbed.

syndrome (ARDS). Such diverse insults as shock, drug injury, aspiration, and bacterial sepsis may provoke a combined problem of lung inflammation, alveolar edema, and pulmonary cell injury. The resulting liberation of many of the potent chemical substances described above are important in creating the end result seen during ARDS, namely, hypoxemia, decreased lung compliance, and pulmonary edema. The interactions among cyclooxygenase and lipoxygenase products from prostaglandin metabolism, as well as the secretions of platelets (serotonin) and alveolar macrophages, all need to be further studied as mediators of acute lung injury.

REACTIVITY OF THE AIRWAYS

A. FIBROUS FRAMEWORK OF THE LUNGS

The entire fibrous interstitium of the lung is interconnected, eventually to the visceral pleura, such that inspiration brings a continual, varying, and interconnected traction on all of this tissue. Thus, the patency of the airways at all stages of a breathing cycle is reasonably ensured.

There are three types of fibers, each with their own physical and chemical properties, and different specific roles in addition to their contribution to this most elaborate supportive framework called the lung interstitium. The *elastic fibers* are the most resilient and distensible. Their primary role is to provide recoil forces that restore smaller airways and vessels to their resting dimensions following inspiration. They can stretch up to twice their length with no structural damage.

Collagen fibers are much less stretchable. Their role is to set the limits of distensibility of the small vessels and alveoli. *Reticular fibers* are most common around smaller blood vessels. They are resistant to stretching, keep the capillary network from excessive dilation, and ensure optimum blood flow to many vessels rather than excessive flow to a few.

When one considers this interstitium in the context of all the other tissue in the lung, one can appreciate the articulate summary statement written by Donald L. Fry and Robert E. Hyatt in their description of pulmonary mechanics, written in 1960: "From a mechanical point of view the lung consists of a large conglomerate of minute expansible air spaces that ventilate to the periphery through a complex arborized pathway. The air spaces and air passages contain fluid surfaces and tissue that possess quasi-elastic properties. For simplicity we may consider all of these elastic elements to act as a continuous three-dimensional elastic mesh ramifying throughout the entire lung parenchyma. During breathing the tension in the 'mesh' increases during inspiration and decreases during expiration."

B. INNERVATION OF THE LUNGS

The caliber of arterioles and bronchioles in the lung can be altered as a result of nervous activity. This area of study has recently gained in importance as the problems of irritant-induced constriction have, in turn, stimulated thinking toward modification of nervous activity by drug manipulation.

Because of an embryological origin similar to the gastrointestinal tract, the smooth muscle and mode of innervation of the two systems are similar. However, it must be realized that great species variation exists regarding the details of innervation. What is true for the human may be quite different in the dog, guinea pig, or rabbit. This discussion will relate to what is known about human airway innervation.

The airways have a sensory (afferent) and a motor (efferent) innervation, and it is primarily via the vagus nerve. Sensory fibers begin in the pulmonary pleura and walls of the bronchi, bronchioles, and alveolar ducts. Some neurons have stretch receptors at their terminal afferent endings, but many remain unmodified, being responsive to noxious agents. Axons of these sensory neurons travel via the vagus nerve to the brainstem, where synaptic connections allow appropriate motor responses. In the instance of lung stretch (during inspiration) the response might be an inhibition of continued lung inflation. Stimulation from noxious substances might elicit bronchoconstriction.

Motor neurons that are part of the vagus nerve extend to airway smooth muscle as well as to tracheal and bronchial glands. When stimulated, they release their stored neurotransmitter chemical, acetylcholine. This substance, when it contacts smooth muscle and glandular cells, will cause bronchoconstriction and glandular secretion, respectively. The response when this vagal (or parasympathetic) activity predominates is termed a "cholinergic" response, named after the neurotransmitter substance acetylcholine.

While parasympathetic innervation to the respiratory tract is well-known and effective, a sympathetic innervation (or "adrenergic" because of the release of the sympathetic neurotransmitter called noradrenaline) is not nearly as defined. Anatomists have discovered considerable species variation in the extent of sympathetic innervation to respiratory tract tissue, and in humans not much is found. In both gastrointestinal and respiratory tract tissue, additional neurons exist, which release a neurotransmitter that probably contains adenosine. The effect of such stimulation is bronchodilation and inhibition of secretions, but other details of this system are lacking. Adenosine is one of a group of organic chemical substances known as purines. Thus, a nervous system response involving adenosine or its related substances as neurotransmitters is termed a purinergic response.

Findings from gastrointestinal pathology suggest how derangements in this pattern of innervation may cause some of the problems observed in diseases such as asthma. In Hirschsprung's disease this purinergic responsiveness is absent, the result being development of a functional spasm of the gastrointestinal tract from uncontrolled parasympathetic stimulation of smooth muscle contraction. The result is a great difficulty in passage of stool. Normally, the purinergic system can inhibit the excitatory effects of acetylcholine, as well as histamine, released by mast cells in diseases such as asthma. Any operational defect in this system may result in loss of control over smooth muscle tension generation. It has been postulated that the hyper-reactive airways observed in chronic bronchitis and asthma may be simply an inability of this purinergic system to exert its normal controlling influence. Considerable investigation is needed in this area. For example, we don't really know where all cell bodies of the purinergic neurons are located.

Smooth muscle obtained from the airways of individuals with respiratory disorders, such as pneumonia and chronic obstructive pulmonary disease, behaves differently from healthy smooth muscle. It is sensitive to norepinephrine, contracting in its presence. Normally, there is little if any response. Thus, something resulting from these disease processes increases the ability of this muscle for its normally present but largely unresponsive adrenergic receptors to respond to adrenergic agents.

There are several types of adrenergic receptors, alpha and beta (β_1 and β_2) being most recognized. These receptor types are variably distributed on smooth and cardiac muscle cell membranes around the body. In the heart, for example, β_1 receptor stimulation increases both the force of cardiac contraction and also the heart rate. Activation of β_2 receptors decreases tension generation in smooth muscle, thus causing both bronchodilation and vasodilation. Because alpha-blocking agents will inhibit the action of norepinephrine on diseased bronchiolar smooth muscle, it is alpha receptors that must be active in this regard.

Norepinephrine also has an effect on β receptors. Figure 5-7 illustrates β_1 receptor function in cardiac muscle, but the same general principles hold true for smooth muscle. Norepinephrine, or β-adrenergic agonists (mimicking agents) bind to the membrane-bound receptor protein adenyl cyclase. This allows enzymatic conversion of ATP within the muscle cell to ADP and cyclic adenosine monophosphate (c-AMP) as shown by the following equation:

$$\text{ATP + Nep (or } \beta\text{-stimulants)} \xrightarrow{\text{Adenyl cyclase}} \text{Cyclic AMP + ADP}$$

Intracellular calcium levels within the smooth muscle cells are regulated in part by c-AMP activity. In bronchiolar smooth muscle it keeps these levels low, thus inhibiting tension generation and yielding bronchodilation. The enzyme phosphodiesterase inactivates c-AMP, so the action of c-AMP is transitory.

Thus, although human airways may not have functional adrenergic innervation, the airway smooth muscle does have the ability to react to adrenergic neurotransmitters. Circulation of these through the bloodstream, or circulation of other alpha-receptor and β-receptor agents, can provoke bronchoconstriction or bronchodilation, depending upon circumstances. Thus understanding of specific disease processes demands a knowledge of the typical changes that might be expected either in the behavior of neurons or in the presence of receptor-influencing chemicals.

C. ALTERATION OF AIRWAY DIAMETER BY PHARMACOLOGIC AGENTS

Pharmacologic manipulation of respiratory tract smooth muscle activity has been of great interest to pulmonary medicine and respiratory therapy. This has been made possible by better understanding of the neuromuscular mechanisms outlined above. A variety of agents are available to treat respiratory disorders, with minimal side effects on cardiovascular function. To understand their actions, one needs to be aware of their specific mode of action as well as the peculiarities of each disease process. A few examples are appropriate here to illustrate the interactive understanding of the disciplines of physiology, pharmacology, and pathology.

Derivatives of xanthine, such as theophylline, inhibit the action of phos-

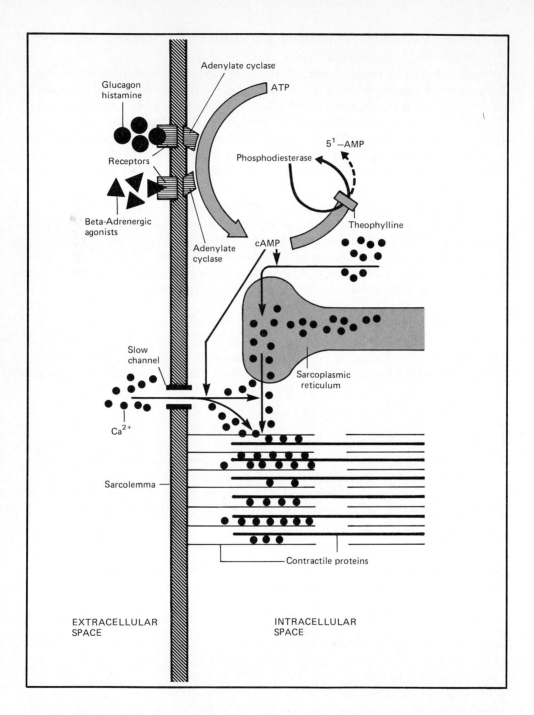

phodiesterase on the hydrolysis of c-AMP (see *Figure 5-7*). These are bronchodilators, since they prolong the effectiveness of c-AMP. Pharmacologic agents such as isoetharine, terbutaline, and metaproterenol will bind specifically to β_2 receptors, thus also causing dilation.

In pulmonary emphysema, the evidence suggests that it is in fact increased parasympathetic activity that causes airway obstruction. (The major problem, of course, is the loss of recoil forces caused by a loss of alveolar septa). Thus, bronchodilation in emphysema may be achieved by use of an appropriate combination of anticholinergic agents (such as atropine) and adrenergic agents, such as the xanthine compounds mentioned above.

Asthma, however, is a more complex disease to understand as well as treat, because of multiple agents in the blood that might initiate bronchoconstriction or vasoconstriction. In particular, there are the constrictors of mast cell origin, namely the leukotrienes and "2" series prostaglandins described earlier. These may actually be the principal initiators of the airway hyperreactivity seen among asthmatic patients. These patients may have epithelial airway cells with a lower-than-normal threshold for pathways of arachidonic acid metabolism, as outlined in *Figure 5-6*.

RELEVANT READING

Austen, K.F. Tissue mast cells in immediate hypersensitivity. *Hospital Practice* **17** (11):98–108, 1982.

Barnes, N.C., and Costello, J.F. Mast-cell-derived mediators in asthma. *Postgraduate Medicine* **76** (5):140–151, 1984.

Bone, R. Adult respiratory distress syndrome. *Seminars in Respiratory Medicine* 8 (Suppl.):1–5, 1986.

Breeze, R.G., and Wheddon, E.B. The cells of the pulmonary airways. *American Review of Respiratory Disease* **116**:705–778, 1977.

Caldwell, P.R.B., Seegal, B.C., Hsu, K.C., Das, M., and Soffer, R.L. Angiotensin-converting enzyme: vascular endothelial localization. *Science* **191**:1050–1051, 1975.

Darin, J. The mode of action of cyclic AMP. Respiratory AMP. *Respiratory Care* **26**:228–240, 1981.

Davies, P. The structure of respiratory defense mechanisms. *Seminars in Respiratory Medicine* 1:221–222, 1980.

Figure 5-7. Diagram of beta receptors in the wall of cardiac muscle (with a similar situation occurring in smooth muscle). Stimulation of the beta receptors by agonist substances (or in cardiac muscle by glucagon or histamine) stimulates the adenylate cyclase enzyme system to increase cellular quantities of cyclic AMP (cAMP) - β_1 receptors are in cardiac muscle, β_2 receptors in bronchiolar and arteriolar smooth muscle. Cyclic AMP levels can be increased also through inhibition of its inactivating enzyme, phosphodiesterase, by xanthine derivatives such as theophylline. Reprinted by permission from *Hospital Practice* **19** (5): 63, 1984.

Dorer, F.E., Kahn, J.R., Lentz, K.E., Levine, M. and Sheggs, L.T. Hydrolysis of bradykinin by angiotensin-converting enzyme. *Circulation Research* **34**:824–827, 1974.

Forrest, J.B. Structural aspects of gas exchange. *Federation Proceedings* **38**:209–214, 1979.

Fry, D.L. and Hyatt, R.E. Pulmonary mechanics. *American Journal of Medicine* **29**:672–689, 1960.

Gail, D.B., and Lenfant, C.J.M. Cells of the lung: biology and clinical implications. *American Review of Respiratory Disease* **127**:366–387, 1983.

Green, G.M., Jahab, G.J., Low, R.B. and Davis, G.S. Defense mechanisms of the respiratory membrane. *American Review of Respiratory Disease* **115**:479–514, 1977.

Gross, N.J., and Skorodin, M.S. Role of the parasympathetic system in airway obstruction due to emphysema. *New England Journal of Medicine* **311**:421–425, 1984.

Hayashi, M. and Huber, G.L. Airway defenses. *Seminars in Respiratory Medicine* **1**:233–239, 1980.

Hinds, W.C. The lung and the environment. *Seminars in Respiratory Medicine* **1**:197–210, 1980.

Hocking, W.G., and Golde, D.W. The pulmonary alveolar macrophage. *New England Journal of Medicine* **301**:580–587, 639–645, 1979.

Huber, G.L. Immunologic lung reactions. *Seminars in Respiratory Medicine* **1**:251–272, 1980.

Huber, G.L., and Davies, P. Alveolar defenses. *Seminars in Respiratory Medicine:* **1**:240–250, 1980.

Huber, G.L. Perspectives: pulmonary host defenses, the host and the development of lung disease. *Seminars in Respiratory Medicine* **1**:187–196, 1980.

Huber, J.F. Practical correlative anatomy of the bronchial tree and lungs. *Journal of the National Medical Association* **41**:49–55, 1949.

Jeffrey, P.K., and Reid, L.M. The respiratory mucus membrane. *In* "Respiratory Defense Mechanisms, Part I," (J.D. Brain, D.F. Proctor, and L.M. Reid, eds.), Marcel Dekker, New York, pp. 193, 1977.

Kuhn, C. Ultrastructure and cellular function of the distal lung. *In* "The Lung: Structure, Function and Disease." (W.M. Thurlbeck, M.R. Abell, eds.), Williams and Wilkins, Baltimore, pp. 1, 1978.

Low, F.N., and Daniels, C.W. Electron microscopy of rat lung. *Anatomical Record* 113:437, 1952.

Megahed, G.E., Senna, G.A., Eissa, M.H., Saleh, S.Z., and Eissa, H.A. Smoking versus infection as the aetiology of mucous gland hypertrophy in chronic bronchitis. *Thorax* **22**:271–278, 1967.

Middleton, E. A rational approach to asthma therapy. *Postgraduate Medicine* **67** (3):107–122, 1980.

Ng, K.K.F., and Vane, J.R. Fate of angiotensin I in the circulation. *Nature* **218**:144–150, 1968.

Orehek, J. Neurohumoral control of airway caliber. *International Review of Physiology* 23:4–74, 1981.

Reid, L. and Jones. R. Bronchial mucosal cells. *Federation Proceedings* **38**:191–196, 1979.

Richardson, J. B., and Ferguson, C.C. Neuromuscular structure and function in the airways. *Federation Proceedings* **38**:202–208, 1979.

Roth, S.H. The emerging new arthritis drugs. *Postgraduate Medicine* **73** (3):125–134, 1983.

Ryan, J.W., and Ryan, U.S. Pulmonary endothelial cells. *Federation Proceedings* 36:2683–2691, 1977.

Ryan, J.W. Processing of endogenous polypeptides by the lungs. *Annual Review of Physiology*, **44**:241–255, 1982.

Said, S.I., The lung in relation to hormones—an update. *Respiratory Care* **26**:660–665, 1981.

Soffer, R.L., Reza, R., and Caldwell, P.R.B. Angiotensin converting enzyme from rabbit pulmonary particles. *Proceedings of the National Academy of Sciences (USA)* **71**:1720–1724, 1974.

Thurlbeck, W.M., and Wang, N. The structure of the lungs. *International Review of Physiology* **2**:1–30, 1974.

Thurlbeck, W.M. Structure of the Lungs. *International Review of Physiology.* **14**:1–36, 1977.

Weibel, E.R., and Gomez, D.M. Architecture of the human lung. *Science* **137**:577–585, 1962.

Weibel, E.R. Morphometry of the human lung. Springer Verlag, Berlin, 1963.

Weiss, J.M. Drazen, J.M., Cole, N. et. al. Bronchoconstrictor effects of leukotriene C in humans. *Science* **216**:196–198, 1982.

Weissmann, G. The eicosanoids of asthma. *New England Journal of Medicine* **308**:454–456, 1983.

Mechanical Aspects of Gas Flow in the Lungs

Chapter Six

Chapter Six Outline

The lungs are deformable organs, set within an expandable but more rigid chest cage. During inspiration or expiration, the lung is distorted from its resting position, and forces tend to bring it back to its resting state. The contributing elements to these forces are many and varied, and include not only the chest cage tissues and pleural membranes, but also the fibrous tissue of the lungs. Gravity changes the manner by which the lungs are inflated and deflated; thus, different postures affect ventilation. As the lungs expand, the pulmonary capillaries become narrower, and the alveolar walls become thinner; the fibrous tissue of the lungs is stretched. Diseased lungs, depending upon the nature of the disease, behave differently during ventilation than healthy lungs, and these differences affect their ability to oxygenate blood and remove CO_2 from it. Thus, it is important to have a good understanding of the dynamics of pulmonary function, especially the importance between proper maintenance of good health and the combination of optimum lung volumes and flow rates. The essence of measuring these parameters is known as pulmonary function testing. This chapter focuses on the highlights of such testing from a functional viewpoint, and introduces the problems of considering the resistance offered from various sources to ensure adequate gas exchange.

MEASUREMENT CONCEPTS FOR PULMONARY FUNCTION TESTING

The term usually applied to the process of assessing lung function is "spirometry," derived from the Latin "spirare" (to breathe) and the Greek "metron" (to measure). The first spirometer was used by Jonathan Hutchinson in 1846, and over the years its importance has equalled the electrocardiograph as a screening mechanism for organ disease. Whereas the electrocardiogram is a record of electrical heart activity, showing possible abnormality, the spirogram is a record of mechanical lung performance also revealing possible abnormality. Modern hospitals now use sophisticated equipment which allows other tests of lung function, but classical spirometry *(Figure 6-1)* still provides information of sufficient diagnostic and therapeutic value that it not only continues to be used side by side with sophisticated hospital technology but also can be used alone effectively in a physician's office.

Good data collection requires therapists who are competent in several areas. First, they must understand the relevant laws of physics, particularly in this context the law of Jacques Charles. When air moves from a region of higher temperature to one of lower temperature, it decreases in volume. Thus, the volume of gas exhaled from the lungs will typically be about 10% larger in the lungs than when it occupies the chamber of the spirometer. A correction must be made to the spirometer volumes (which are at ambient temperature and pressure, saturated, or ATPS), to make them more nearly equal to lung volumes (which are at body temperature and pressure, or BTPS). Table 6-1 gives the necessary

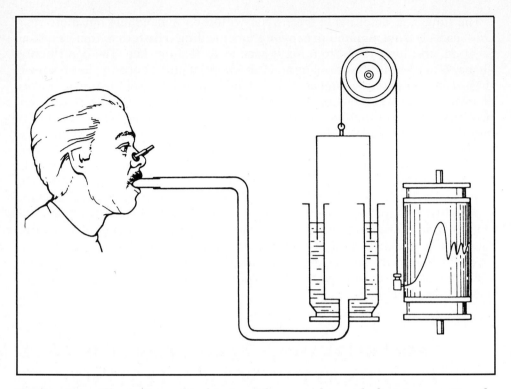

Figure 6-1.   Illustration of subject, with nose clamped shut to permit only mouth breathing, exhaling into the bell of a water-sealed spirometer. Increased volume of air into the bell raises it, causing a downward deflection of the recording pen on the adjacent kymograph. Performance of specific breathing maneuvers allows determination of certain lung volumes, capacities, and flow rates.

information for making such corrections. As an example, a tidal volume measurement of 450 ml ATPS, obtained when the room temperature was 22°C, would convert to 491 ml BTPS (450 ml × 1.091).

Second, therapists must be skillful in acquiring objectively useful data. When maximum volumes or flow rates are to be assessed, the subject must in fact deliver an all-out effort. Even when testing sedentary healthy people or athletes, this involves more than proper instructions and good-natured encouragement. With patients for whom breathing of any sort is difficult or painful, far more is required of a competent therapist. It requires a positive frame of mind—the desire to perform well for the therapist on the part of the subject tested, and a great desire on the part of the therapist to properly evaluate. There must be reproducibility in the data obtained—no leaks in the equipment system, and uniformly proper subject breathing efforts. Repeat performance of these effort-dependent maneuvers must yield good duplication if conclusions based upon the data are to characterize pulmonary limitations accurately.

TABLE 6-1.   Conversion of ATPS Gas Volumes, Obtained from Spirometry, to BTPS Volumes.

Factor to Convert Vol. to 37°C Sat.	When Gas Temperature (C) Is	With Water Vapor Pressure (Mm Hg) of
1.102	20	17.5
1.096	21	18.7
1.091	22	19.8
1.085	23	21.1
1.080	24	22.4
1.075	25	23.8
1.068	26	25.2
1.063	27	26.7
1.057	28	28.3
1.051	29	30.0
1.045	30	31.8
1.039	31	33.7
1.032	32	35.7
1.026	33	37.7
1.020	34	39.9
1.014	35	42.2
1.007	36	44.6
1.000	37	47.0

LUNG VOLUMES AND CAPACITIES, AND THEIR SIGNIFICANCE

The lung has four definable volumes, illustrated in *Figure 6-2*. The amount of air inspired or expired during quiet breathing is called *tidal volume* (TV), and in a 70 kilogram healthy man this averages 500 ml. Actually only about 350 ml of this volume reaches the alveoli. The other 150 ml, approximating the individual's ideal body weight in pounds, remains in the conducting space of the nose, pharynx, larynx, trachea, and bronchi, and is termed *anatomic dead space* because it plays no role in gas exchange with the blood. This will be discussed further in Chapter Eight.

We have the ability to inspire considerably more than 500 ml of air. This volume is logically termed the *inspiratory reserve volume* (IRV). It is the additional volume of air that can be inspired following a typical tidal volume inhalation. Correspondingly, there is a volume of air that can be expired following a typical tidal volume exhalation. This is the *expiratory reserve volume* (ERV).

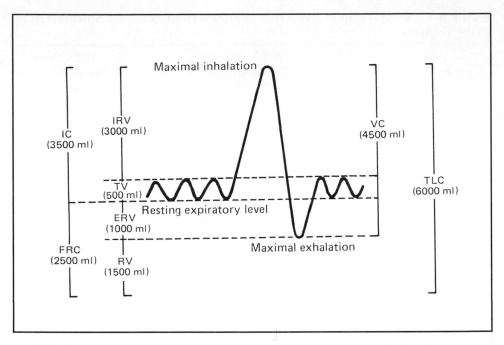

Figure 6-2.   Lung volumes and capacities. The sum of residual volume (RV), expiratory reserve volume (ERV), inspiratory reserve volume (IRV), and tidal volume (TV) equals the total capacity of the lung (TLC). The amount of air inhalable following a normal exhalation is the inspiratory capacity (IC), whereas the total amount inhalable following a maximum exhalation is the vital capacity (VC). That amount of air remaining in the lungs following a normal exhalation is the functional residual capacity (FRC).

From Youtsey, J.W. "Basic Pulmonary Function Measurements", *Egan's Fundamentals of Respiratory Therapy,* 4th Ed., C.B. Spearman, Ed., St. Louis, C.V. Mosby Co., 1982.

Even following expiration of all the air accessible voluntarily (IRV + TV + ERV = 3,000 + 500 + 1,000 = 4,500 ml), still another 1,500 ml remains in the lungs because the lower intrathoracic pressure keeps the alveoli slightly inflated. This is the *residual volume* (RV). Opening the thoracic cavity allows equilibration of intrathoracic with atmospheric pressure, and this RV would exit, leaving a very small volume remaining in the essentially collapsed lungs.

Medico-legally the residual volume is significant. Fetal and stillborn lungs contain no air; hence, a piece of their lung tissue will not float in water. A piece of lung from a baby born live but who subsequently died will indeed float because it has been inflated.

Lung capacities are calculated by combining at least two lung volumes *(Figure 6-2). Inspiratory capacity* (IC) indicates the total inspiratory ability of the lungs, beginning from the end expiratory position, and is the sum of the tidal and inspiratory reserve volumes (3,500 ml). The *functional residual capacity* (FRC) is the sum of the residual and expiratory reserve volumes (2,500 ml) and represents the gas remaining in the lungs at the end-expiratory position. This amount of air will be used for exchange with the pulmonary capillary blood before the next inspiration begins. The *vital capacity* (VC) is the sum of three volumes: inspiratory reserve, expiratory reserve, and tidal (3,000 + 1,000 + 500 = 4,500 ml). Finally, the *total lung capacity* (TLC) is the sum of all lung volumes, thus adding residual volume to the vital capacity (6,000 ml). Via spirometry, neither the RV nor the FRC or TLC can be measured. However, these lung compartments can be determined simply and accurately by plethysmography *(Figure 6-3)*.

These volume and capacities are static measurements, and indicate different levels of lung expansion that typically should be attainable. There are three important factors that change these static lung volumes. One is age. As one grows older, there is a decrease in the elastic recoil of the lungs, and an increase in the stiffness of the thoracic cage. This shifts the end-expiratory position upward, thereby increasing the FRC. With age there is a gradual shift upward toward a decreased VC and IRV, an increased RV and FRC, with TV unchanged. The aging process can be partly offset by a vigorous exercising lifestyle. While not increasing one's lifespan, the elevated physical activity over a lifetime slows the rate of lung/chest degeneration.

Another factor is body size. Values for men and women are different at any given age because of mean differences in body size. Within either sex, at any given age, taller individuals tend to have larger lung volumes, but racial variations occur as well. Blacks normally have smaller lung volumes than whites, for example, explained perhaps by a tendency for a smaller thoracic cage and longer lower limb length caused by long thigh bones.

A third factor is posture. As one moves from a seated, upright position to the supine position, the FRC decreases, and VC may decrease as well. When seated upright and breathing easily, our lungs are about 50% inflated at the end-expiratory position, but this reduces to 33% in the supine position.

Despite all these constraints and sources of variation, which have been accounted for through the construction of tables of comparison and normal testing protocols, abnormal values for volumes and capacities can be distinguished rather easily and consistently. Such abnormalities suggest any of several diseases or conditions that might limit the expansibility of the lungs or thoracic cage. As a group they are termed restrictive lung diseases. However, it should be emphasized that one can have many of these volume and capacity parameters essentially unchanged from normal while still manifesting the early stages of restrictive disease. No one of these parameters is diagnostic by itself, except for TLC, which may be decreased with restrictive lung diseases and elevated in obstructive lung diseases. However, TLC can be normal in early obstructive diseases or in between asthma exacerbations.

The limitations to lung expansibility are many and varied, and are outlined in Table 6-2. Although spirometric evaluation by itself does not allow diagnoses of problems such as those listed, it does allow assessment of the extent of each

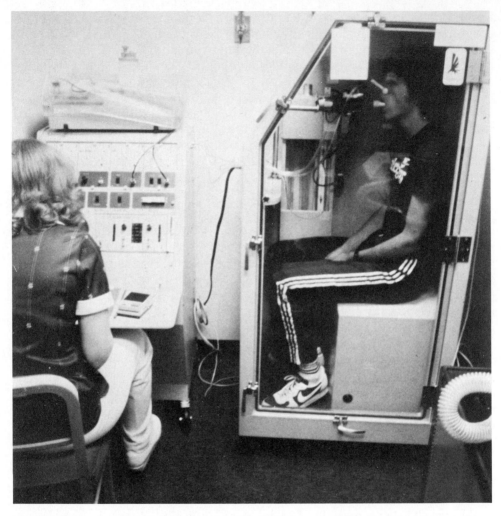

Figure 6-3. A subject seated in a body plethysmograph, used to measure lung volumes not accessible with spirometry. The chamber is sealed, and chamber pressure is measured using sensitive pressure transducers. The subject breathes, with thoracic volume changes being sensed within the chamber. Airway pressure can be measured at various thoracic volumes by closing a shutter that occludes the airway. (Photograph courtesy of David E. Martin).

functional disturbance, and long-term monitoring of the course of recovery or progression of impairment.

LUNG FLOW RATES AND
THEIR SIGNIFICANCE

Just as important as lung volumes is the quickness (implying ease) with which the lungs can inflate and deflate. Disturbances in the ease with which air moves

Table 6-2. Limitations to Lung Expansibility

1) Limitation of Respiratory Movements
   a. Muscular Dystrophy
   b. Neuromusclar Junction Problems
   c. Poliomyelitis
   d. Myasthenia Gravis
   e. Depression of Central Respiratory Centers
2) Limitation of Thoracic Cage Expansion
   a. Body Deformities such as Kyphoscoliosis
   b. Fractured Ribs
   c. Massive Obesity
   d. Fibrothorax (Calcified Pneumothorax or Emphysema)
3) Limitations of Lung Expansibility
   a. Lung Cysts or Tumors
   b. Pneumothorax
   c. Pleural Effusion
4) Limitations of Diaphragm Movement
   a. Ascites
   b. Pregnancy
   c. Phrenic Nerve Dysfunction
5) Limitation of Quantity of Lung Tissue Available
   a. Surgical Lobectomy
   b. Surgical Pneumonectomy
   c. Bronchial Obstruction with Postobstructive Atelectasis
6) Pain
   a. Pleurisy
   b. Recovering Incision Site from Surgery
   c. Injured Ribs
   d. Costochrondritis

through the respiratory passageways manifest themselves as impaired lung flow rates. All the possible causes of such impaired flow rates are grouped together under the category of obstructive lung diseases. Thus, effective protocols for testing flow dynamics have also evolved as an integral part of spirometry.

If a subject achieves a maximal expiratory effort following a maximal inspiratory effort, but now as quickly as possible—under the constraints of time—a *forced vital capacity* (FVC) curve is obtained, illustrated in *Figure 6-4*. Its magnitude as measured in liters, should be similar to one obtained under less forceful conditions. As seen in *Figure 6-4*, after about 4 seconds of forced exhalation, a FVC value of about 5 liters is measured. This tracing was produced on a rapidly moving sheet of paper, allowing the quantitation of how much air was exhaled during each second of forced exhalation. Thus, a *forced expiratory volume* can be determined for each full second following the onset of exhalation ($FEV_{1.0}$, $FEV_{2.0}$, $FEV_{3.0}$, and so on).

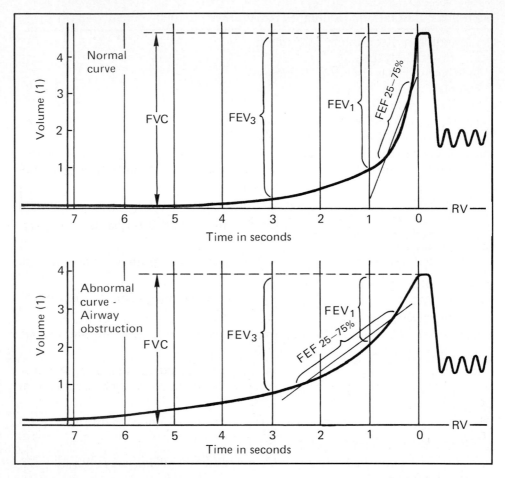

Figure 6-4. Estimating lung flow rates and forced vital capacity (FVC). Following a maximum inhalation, the subject exhales maximally, allowing FVC determination. Use of a rapidly moving paper recording system spreads this activity such that the forced expiratory volume can be calculated for periods such as one second (FEV1), two seconds (FEV2), etc. The forced midexpiratory flow rate between the points where 25% and 75% of the FEV has occurred is determined by calculating the slope of the line (L/sec) connecting the 25% and 75% points.

From Youtsey, J.W. "Basic Pulmonary Function Measurements", *Egan's Fundamentals of Respiratory Therapy*, 4th Ed., C.B. Spearman, Ed., St. Louis, C.V. Mosby Co., 1982.

Another commonly-used method for expressing this is to divide $FEV_{1.0}$ by FVC and multiply by 100, normally expressing $FEV_{1.0}$ as a percent of FVC. Thus, $(FEV_{1.0}/FVC) \times 100 = 80\%$. Although not depicted in *Figure 6-4*, the FEV for one half sec is often measured (represented as $FEV_{0.5}$). Typically, $(FEV_{.5}/FVC) \times 100 = 50\%$ of FVC, and $(FEV_1/FVC) \times 100 = 70–85\%$ of FVC. Active young healthy adults may do much better than this and may expire all of their FVC by

2.5 to 3 seconds, in contrast to the more usual 3–4 seconds in sedentary people.

Flow rates during various periods of the maximum forced exhalation described by the FVC curve can be measured easily. Provided that the measuring instrument itself has very low resistance to airflow, the results will indicate the ability of the chest-lung system to move air. The flow rate over the middle portion of the expiratory curve is the least effort-dependent. Thus, a reduction in this measured variable is a sensitive indicator of small-airway obstruction, assuming normal FVC, $FEV_{1.0}$, and $FEV_{1.0}$/FVC ratio.

One quantitative assessment technique is to measure the *forced expiratory flow* during the middle 50% of the FVC maneuver, as shown in *Figure 6-4*. This is done by drawing a straight line through two points representing 25% and 75% of FVC. Then, the line is extended through two one-second time markers. By determining the slope of that line (the number of liters of air flowing per second), the value obtained is the mid-expiratory flow, and referred to as $FEV_{25\%-75\%}$. When assessing the likelihood of small-airway obstructive disease, it is generally accepted that both $FEV_{3.0}$ and $FEF_{25\%-75\%}$ should be significantly decreased from normal values.

A related determination often made is that of *peak expiratory flow rate* (PEFR), the maximum flow occurring over the most rapidly changing portion of the FVC curve. Normally this occurs at its very beginning, where flows may average 9 to 10 liters per second.

Another common measurement, but requiring a different maneuver, is the *maximum voluntary ventilation* (MVV), sometimes termed the *maximum breathing capacity* (MBC). The subject breathes as rapidly and effectively as possible for 12 to 15 seconds. The total volume of air expelled is quantified. Normally, this is 160 to 180 L/min, but because of its relative nonspecificity and great dependence on effort, only large deviations from predicted values have clinical significance. In trained athletes, however, for whom such maneuvers as MVV and PEFR determination represent a performance challenge, the variability among repeat determinations diminishes greatly. Among endurance runners, for example, comparison of MVV (in liters per minute) with expired ventilation ($\dot{V}_E$) values (also in liters/minute) at maximum performance (during ergometer or treadmill stress testing) provides a means for assessing the extent of ventilatory limitation at those high work rates.

The advent of electronic devices in spirometry has brought with it new methods of presenting data, some of which have had useful clinical relevance. One such device allows the construction of a *flow volume loop* by having the subject perform first a maximum forced expiration from TLC to RV, followed by a maximum forced inspiration back to TLC. *Figure 6-5* illustrates three such loops. An X-Y recorder is used to graph flow (on the ordinate) and volume (on the abscissa) simultaneously. Expiration is described above the horizontal line representing zero flow, inspiration below it. Both TLC and RV positions are indicated on the zero-flow line. Starting at the asterisked TLC position, the arrows trace the formation of these curves. Using this graphic presentation, peak expiratory and inspiratory flows are easily identified, as well as FVC. $FEF_{25\%-75\%}$ can also be determined, as indicated. The lowered lung volume measurements in patients with restrictive disease, and the decreased lung volume as well as flow ratio measurements in patients with obstructive disease, show up well in flow-volume loop assessment.

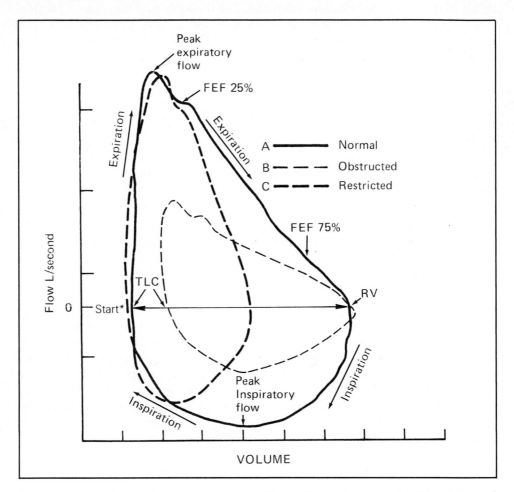

Figure 6-5. Flow volume loops created by subjects who are healthy (A), and with obstructive (B) or restrictive (C) lung disease. Beginning at the asterisked point, the curves are created as subjects move from TLC through maximum expiration (upward, then downward) to RV, where zero flow occurs for a brief moment before maximum inspiration to TLC occurs (downward, then upward), returning to the starting point. From this loop, peak flows, FVC, and FEF$_{25\%-75\%}$ are also easily determined.

Examples of obstructive lung disease include bronchitis, pulmonary emphysema, asthma, and bronchiectasis. There may be bronchospasm, edema, or tenacious mucus secretions, or loss of small airway integrity. Because of the increased airway obstruction, air flow rates will be reduced due to the greater intrathoracic pressure required, but not conveniently generated. A decrease in flow at the end of expiration implies small airway obstruction, but at the beginning it implies large airway obstruction.

Cigarette smoking is a cause of two major obstructive lung diseases—pulmonary emphysema and chronic bronchitis. Cessation of smoking during the early stages of these diseases can limit their progression. For this reason the test of $FEF_{25\%-75\%}$ is highly regarded, for it can detect early signs of obstruction. Presently, the death rate from chronic obstructive pulmonary diseases is half that of lung cancer, which makes it a major health problem. Many more people will develop chronic bronchitis and pulmonary emphysema than lung cancer from cigarette smoking. The debilitation of lifestyle is enormous, because of the increased severity of upper respiratory infections, raising the total number of days missed from work.

CAUTIONS AND PROBLEMS
WITH SPIROMETRY

A few methodological cautions for collecting data have already been mentioned. Because of the myriad of pathologies that can occur, interpretation of data may not always be straightforward. For example, some patients have obstructive and restrictive problems simultaneously. Consider the chronic cigarette smoker who is also very obese, or the patient with pulmonary emphysema who has only one lung. The possibilities are almost endless.

When performing spirometry, one must be aware of any personal problems that might alter the ability to obtain accurate results. Certain medications, emotional problems, weakness, pain, allergic reactions, and recent respiratory ailments unrelated to the patient's primary problem all can compromise meaningful data collection.

Normally, results of spirometric tests are reported as a percent of a normal predicted value. However, various nomograms and regression equations are also available for estimating normal spirometric values for both men and women simply on the basis of age, sex, and body height. A nomogram is an arrangement of two or more graduated lines constituting scales of values, whereby, from two known values, a third can be readily determined. Those of Morris, Koski, and Johnson, illustrated in Figure 6-6, are frequently used for FVC, $FEF_{25\%-75\%}$ and $FEV_{1.0}$. As an example, notice the line drawn through points representing a 68 inch tall, 40-year-old male in Figure 6-6. One would estimate his $FEV_{1.0}$ as 3.7 L, and his $FEF_{25\%-75\%}$ as 3.9 L/sec.

It should be realized however, that nomograms of this sort may not always be completely reliable. There is, of course, the need to be precise in connecting data points. Even then, there are unique situations that can also give errors in the use of such nomograms. For example, these predicted nomographic values should be

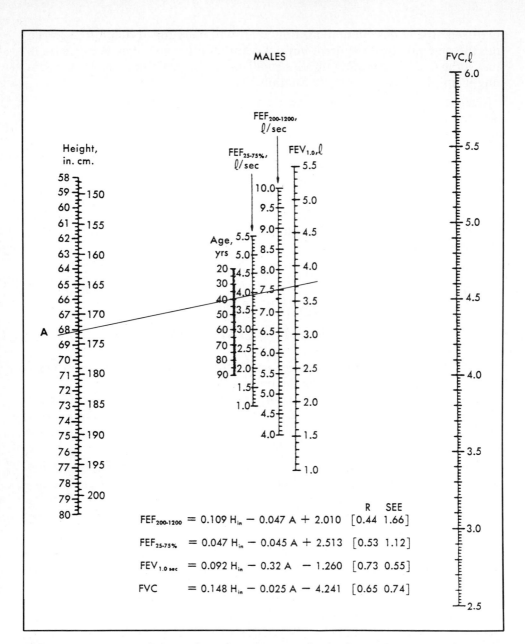

Figure 6-6. One of several nomograms available for estimating pulmonary function parameters. These illustrated here, developed by Morris, Koski, and Johnson, allow estimation of FVC, FEF, and FEV. (Reprinted with permission from *American Review of Respiratory Disease* 103:57–67, 1971.

reduced by 15% for black males, but not for black females; black males differ from white males in this important respect. Also, in kyphoscoliosis patients one should use total horizontal arm span instead of body height because of the

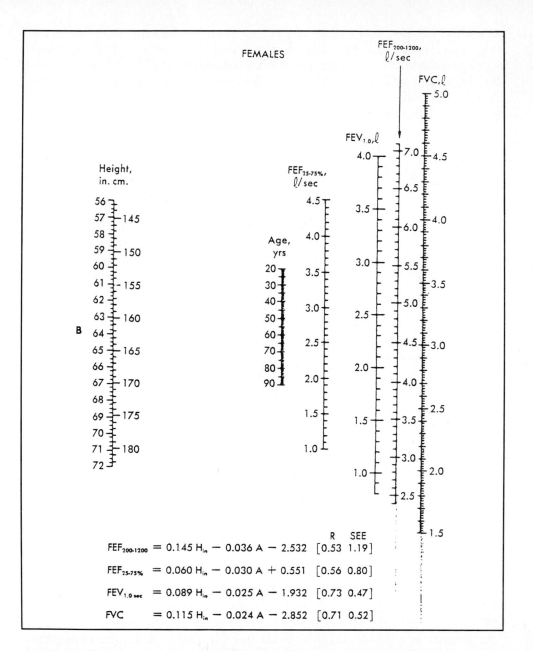

FEMALES

FEF$_{200-1200,}$ ℓ/sec

FVC, ℓ

Height,
in. cm.

FEF$_{25-75\%,}$ ℓ/sec

FEV$_{1.0,}$ℓ

Age,
yrs

	R	SEE
FEF$_{200-1200}$ = 0.145 H$_{in}$ − 0.036 A − 2.532	[0.53	1.19]
FEF$_{25-75\%}$ = 0.060 H$_{in}$ − 0.030 A + 0.551	[0.56	0.80]
FEV$_{1.0 sec}$ = 0.089 H$_{in}$ − 0.025 A − 1.932	[0.73	0.47]
FVC = 0.115 H$_{in}$ − 0.024 A − 2.852	[0.71	0.52]

measurement inaccuracies caused from curvature and crookedness of the spine.

Even the comparison of measured results to predicted results can be subject to error. One must ensure, for example, that the measurement procedure for collecting the subject data is the same as that used by the investigators who collected the normative data against which the prediction comparison will be made.

Finally, it should be emphasized that if one attempts always to consider values for the various lung volumes and flow rates from the perspective of how these are generated physiologically, then one is best prepared to explain abnormalities meaningfully. For example, one tends to identify a reduced FEF with well developed obstructive lung disease. If there is a restrictive defect so far advanced that the patient simply cannot force much air through the respiratory tract, then the FEF, normally a clue to obstructive disease, will be reduced in this patient with restrictive disease.

PLEURAL MEMBRANES AND THE SUBATMOSPHERIC INTRAPLEURAL PRESSURE

An important aspect of pulmonary mechanics is the extent to which lung volumes change when pressures of varying magnitude are applied to the lung/chest system. This system behaves somewhat like a spring—it must be stretched during inspiration by the respiratory muscles, and then with expiration, recoil occurs.

Understanding how inspiratory muscle activity can enlarge the thoracic cage is a rather simple task, since the muscles attach to the cage. Understanding how the lungs enlarge requires review of pleural membrane anatomy. As the lungs grow during embryonic life, they invaginate into a closed pleural sac (Figure 6-7). As growth occurs, the portion of pleural membrane in contact with the lung covers its outer surface and even dips into the fissures between its lobes. This is the visceral or pulmonary pleura. Gradually the fluid filling each pleural sac is removed, except for a few milliliters of a serous fluid that remains for lubrication of the now-enlarged lungs. These lungs rub against the inner surface of the chest wall, diaphragm, and structures occupying the middle of the thorax—all covered by pleural membrane as well (the parietal portion).

Thus the pleural sacs essentially disappear, leaving only a potential pleural cavity. The visceral and parietal pleura are continuous with each other around and below the root of the lungs. Movement of the thorax leads to movement of the lung via this pleural membrane linkage, aided by the thin film of lubricating liquid at the interface. Because of the ease in sliding the visceral pleura over the parietal pleura, downward movement of the diaphragm, when it generates tension, enlarges all lobes of the lungs, even if the thorax is fixed.

In normal health, the volume of pleural fluid present at any moment is extremely small, perhaps 3–5 ml, with an alkaline pH of about 7.64. However, this volume can increase dramatically with exercise, up to as much as 30 ml. There is a sizable turnover of pleural fluid each day, between 5 and 10 liters. Filtration of fluid out of the arterial end of the parietal pleural capillaries produces it, and the majority is reabsorbed at the venous end of the visceral pleural capillaries. Any excess filtration is handled by the pleural lymphatic vessels. An excess buildup of fluid in this space is called pleural effusion.

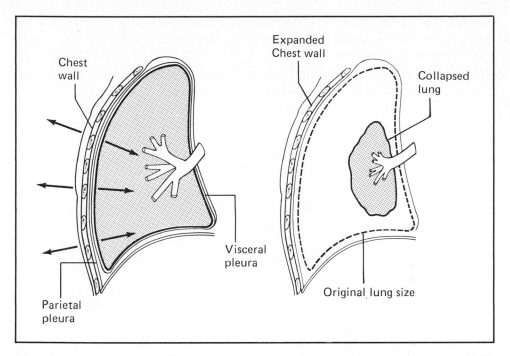

Figure 6-7. Diagram to illustrate the parietal pleura, adherent to the chest wall, and the visceral pleura, adherent to the lungs. Invagination of the embryonic lungs into each pleural sac, and enlargement with subsequent development, eventually fills the pleural cavities except for only a small fluid-filled pleural space. This fluid provides lubrication as the lungs (with their pleural lining) move against the rib cage (with its pleural lining) during breathing. Collapse of a lung, as with a knife wound, increases the volume of the pleural space.

This balancing of several fluid pressures in the pleural membranes is only one example of a similar phenomenon occurring all over the body. The British physiologist Ernest Starling first described this near-equilibrium state around the turn of the century. In health, the fluid filtering out of the circulatory system from the arterial ends of the capillaries is virtually matched by the quantity of fluid resorbed back into the circulation at the venous end. It isn't perfect, and a small net outflow occurs, normally no more than about 3.5 ml/min for the entire body. This excess fluid is returned to the circulation via lymphatic channels. Starling attempted to identify and quantify all the various forces responsible for this ongoing net outflow of fluid from the circulatory system. Blood pressure, of course, is one contributing factor. Another is the osmotic pressure caused by proteins in the plasma and interstitial fluid. Plasma protein osmotic pressure (called oncotic pressure) is typically greater than interstitial osmotic pressure. Water tends to move into the plasma due to oncotic pressure, and into the interstitial space due to interstitial osmotic pressure. Any disruption among these various forces will promote fluid buildup in the interstitial space (edema), or a decrease in lymphatic flow. An equivalent accumulation of fluid buildup in the intrapleural space causes pleural effusion. Such accumulation in the abdominal cavity is termed ascites.

The osmotic pressure relationships caused by protein impermeability explains how pleural effusion can occur when blood pressure is normal. Pleural fluid normally contains very little protein; it is similar to cerebrospinal fluid in this regard. Bacterial or viral pneumonia can cause pleural effusion as a result of inflammation of the adjacent pleural membrane. This inflammation increases membrane permeability to protein, and an increased pleural fluid protein concentration results. This raises the pleural fluid osmotic pressure, and water tends to move into the intrapleural space.

The pressure in the intrapleural space is subatmospheric, averaging 4 to 5 cm H_2O (0.4–0.5 kPa). If air would be introduced into this space, the visceral and parietal layers of pleura would separate. This condition is termed a *pneumothorax*. The lung and thoracic cage would assume new positions, the lungs collapsing because of their elastic recoil, the chest enlarging for the same reason (*Figure 6-7*). Clearly, a balance of forces exists between the two tissues, at the resting or end-expiratory position, and at other points in the ventilatory cycle as well. This balance is determined by the ventilatory muscle tension generated at that moment in the cycle and by the balance between the two recoil forces, i.e., those of the thorax and lung.

There must be a mechanism to prevent respiratory gases from accumulating in the pleural space, since the pleural membranes are indeed permeable to them. The gas pressure in the arterial blood is about 7.5 mmHg (1 kPa) lower than atmospheric because of the inability for O_2 to fully equilibrate. The binding of O_2 and CO_2 to hemoglobin lowers the total venous blood gas pressure to about 53 mmHg (7 kPa) below atmospheric. The slow movement of O_2 from blood into tissues makes the interstitial fluid (and hence pleural fluid) gradient even higher than 7 kPa. Thus, the net direction of diffusion of gases is from interstitial (and pleural) fluid into the bloodstream. This continual gradient keeps the pleural space essentially gas free.

RESISTANCES TO AIRFLOW DURING BREATHING

One ventilatory cycle consists of an inspiration and an expiration (*Figure 6-8*). At two points in this continuum (A, C), there will be zero airflow, i.e., when inspiration and expiration have been completed. At both of these moments intra-alveolar pressure equals ambient (atmospheric) pressure.

At the resting end-expiratory position (A), the recoil of the lung and chest wall are equal and opposite; no air flows and the respiratory muscles are not actively changing their tension. All along the tracheobronchial tree atmospheric pressure prevails. Activation of the inspiratory muscles results in chest expansion (B).

This enlargement of the thoracic cage also increases total intra-alveolar volume, reducing intra-alveolar pressure. Air moves in passively through inspiration, and airflow ceases as inspiration is completed (C). Expiration, being passive in that no muscles actively generate tension (at least, none during resting quiet breathing), allows lung recoil forces to dominate. The lungs diminish in volume, and during this reduction intra-alveolar pressure exceeds atmospheric.

Depending upon the extent of inflation of the lung or enlargement of the chest, greater or lesser resistance to movement will occur. We may define resistance as the opposition to motion caused by the forces of friction. Friction dissipates mechanical energy as heat. This friction is produced by movement of the chest/lung tissues and movement of air through the tracheobronchial tree. Energy must be supplied through action of the respiratory muscles to overcome this resistance. Mathematically, resistance is the rate of flow in response to a given applied pressure.

Actually, resistance takes three forms. There is *inertial resistance*, minimal in the human system, offered by non-moving gases and tissues that must begin to move at various points in any ventilatory cycle. There is *elastic resistance*, developed in the chest/lung tissues whenever a volume change occurs. Some elastic forces in the chest tissues tend to expand the chest, while opposing elastic forces in the lungs tend to deflate the lungs. Thus, during a normal inspiration, the elastic work needed to inflate the chest/lung system is actually less than that required to inflate the lungs alone. During a normal expiration, the elastic energy gained by the lung tissue is transferred without loss to the chest.

With greater inhalation, the elastic forces of the chest/lung system begin to act in the same direction. Considerable energy is required to overcome both. Thus, the optimal frequency for breathing becomes that which leads to adequate ventilation with the least energy cost. Elastic work is inversely related to frequency, i.e., the slower the frequency, the less is the friction, thus the elastic work. At rest we optimize by taking only about a dozen breaths per minute, each reasonably large. This self-adjusting occurs at all work loads. Studies of competitive runners have been particularly interesting in this regard. In a long distance race, they typically take about 192 footstrikes per minute, synchronizing their breathing with one inspiration and expiration for every two footstrikes. This is called a 2:2 pattern, giving a respiratory rate of 48 breaths per minute. As they begin to accumulate more lactic acid in their tissues, thereby increasing the stimulus to breathe, their pattern may switch to a 2:1 ratio, with a faster exhalation. Their cadence will remain remarkably constant, giving them now an elevation in ventilation to 64 breaths per minute. A 1:1 pattern (96 breaths per minute) would not be optimal for sustained gas exchange in view of the nearly doubled volume of nonfunctional (dead space) gas volume moved.

Finally, there is *flow resistance*, offered by the airways as gas moves through them. There are two distinct types of airflow, laminar and turbulent. The resistance to flow depends greatly on what type is involved. *Figure 6-9* illustrates these two types of flow. Laminar flow is characterized by parallel, smoothly sliding layers (or laminae) of liquid or gas. Such flow occurs in airways or tubing

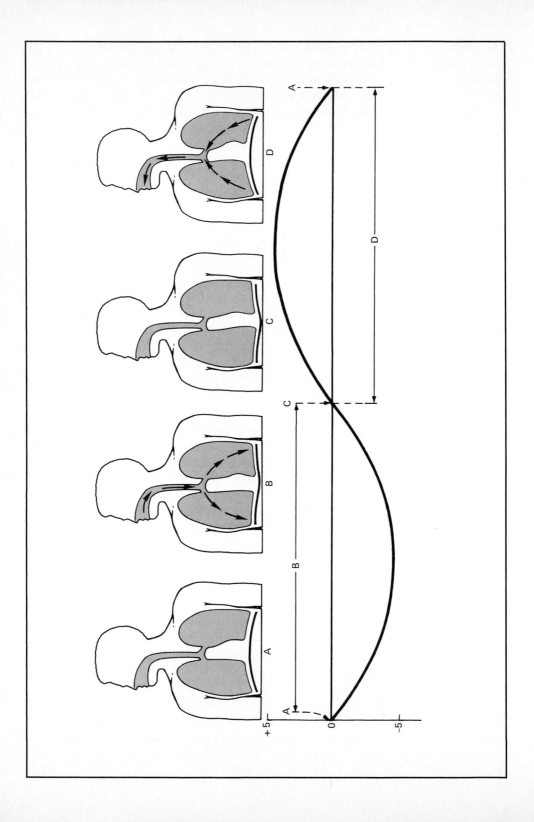

where diameter and direction are constant, or with only minor obstructions or directional alterations. A turbulent flow pattern is a disorderly movement of gas in many directions causing eddies and counter-movements.

If the fluid or gas flow is laminar, then the basic factors determining the resistance to flow (R) are described by Poiseuille's equation. The factors include length of the tube down which flow is occurring (l, in cm), the viscosity of the flowing substance (v, in poises, or dyne-sec/cm^2), and the radius of the tube, (r, in cm). the relationship is given by

$$R = \frac{8 \ln}{\pi r^4}, \text{ in dyne-sec/cm}^5$$

It is clear that the most important factor in this relationship is the vessel radius. A decrease in radius (vasoconstriction or bronchoconstriction) by 50% causes a 16-fold increase in flow resistance. Resistance in the airways is increased during asthma attacks because of bronchoconstriction. It is usually increased during pulmonary emphysema because many airways collapse during exhalation as a result of diminished traction on these vessels from inadequate supporting connective tissue.

Pressure (P) generating flow of blood or air, the quantity of flow ($\dot{Q}$) resulting and the resistance to flow (R) are all related by the relationship:

$$\dot{Q} = \frac{P}{R}, \text{ or } R = \frac{P}{\dot{Q}}, \text{ or } P = \dot{Q}R$$

Thus, by substituting $8 \ln/\pi r^4$ for R, we can write:

$$P = \frac{\dot{Q} \, 8 \ln}{\pi r^4}, \text{ or } V = \frac{\dot{Q} \, \pi \, r^4}{8\ln}$$

While the most important physical property of the vessel or airway during laminar flow is the conduit radius, the most important physical property of the fluid or gas is its viscosity. This is because intermolecular friction is important in sliding flow layers. Table 6-3 compares the viscosity and density of several gases.

The pressure-flow relationship in turbulent flow is dramatically different from that of laminar flow—it is non-linear. Density is now an important physical factor of the fluid. A small increase in flow requires a geometric increase in pressure, since essentially $P = R V^2$ and $R = P/V^2$. Large pressure increases will yield only small flow increases if the flow is turbulent. Thus the work required for maintaining turbulent flow at a given rate is greater than that required for laminar flow.

Figure 6-8. One ventilatory cycle. Starting with zero airflow, at the end-expiratory position (A), air flows into the respiratory tract and lungs upon activation of the inspiratory muscles (B). At the termination of inspiration, and just before expiration, again zero air flow occurs (C). Then, expiration occurs (D) as the inspiratory muscles relax and return the system to its original 'resting' or end-expiratory position (A).

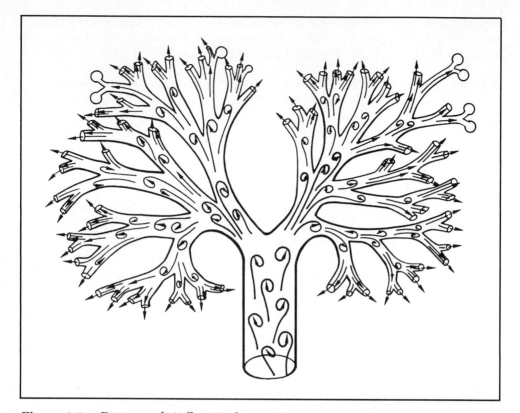

Figure 6-9. Patterns of air flow in the respiratory system. Two types—turbulent and laminar—occur, determined primarily by vessel radius, but affected also by factors such as air pressure, sudden directional changes, and viscosity of the air. In large vessels, with high velocity flow, turbulence often occurs, and this typically also occurs at vessel bifurcations and other sites of sudden directional change. Eddy currents occur, which make the flow more energy costly. Along smaller vessels in the lung, where flow is slow, it is laminar, or streamlined, and energy efficient.

The causes of turbulence can be quantified by Thomas Reynold's equation, which states that $N_R = 2 \rho \bar{v} r/\pi \eta$. Here N_R = Reynold's number, ρ = density in gm/cc^3, $\bar{v}$ = mean velocity in cc/sec, r = radius in cm, and η = viscosity in poises. When N_R exceeds 1,000 to 2,000 (depending upon authors, e.g., Nunn versus Comroe), some turbulence occurs in what at lower values had been laminar flow. Thus, increasing the velocity, increasing the diameter of a tube, or pressurizing the gas may all lead to turbulence. Table 6-4 gives estimates of Reynold's numbers for different portions of the tracheobronchial tree and upper airway, at different flow rates.

Even an introductory knowledge of the common respiratory disease processes will allow recall of examples of clinical situations or disease mechanisms where

TABLE 6–3   Density and Viscosity of Gases Commonly Encountered in Respiratory Physiology

Gas	Viscosity Poises 0°C	Density gm/L @ 760 mmHg
CO_2	142	1.9769
CO	166	1.2504
He	186	0.17847
H	83.5	0.08988
N_2	—	1.2568
O_2	189	1.42904

resistance to airflow could be significantly increased. One clinical situation would be intubation. Certain diseases may increase bronchoconstriction by either nervous or chemical mechanisms, or increase production of bronchial secretions. Vascular mucosal congestion and pulmonary edema will also compromise air flow. Under these circumstances of reduced airway diameter, air flow in a great many lung vessels will almost always be turbulent. In smaller airways, because of their vast numbers, the airflow in any one of them is insufficient to cause turbulence except at vessel branchings where local eddy currents can induce turbulence. However, mucus accumulation or tumors can distort the otherwise uniform diameter of these small vessels, causing turbulent flow as air rushes past narrow, partially blocked regions.

TABLE 6–4.   Reynold's Numbers for Various Regions of the Tracheo-Bronchial Tree*

Location	Diameter mm	Velocity 6 L/min	Velocity 60 L/min	Velocity 200 L/min
Nasal canal	5	400	4,000	12,000
Pharynx	12	800	8,000	24,000
Glottis	8	1,600	16,000	48,000
Trachea	21	1,250	12,500	37,000
Bronchi	17	910	9,100	27,300
Bronchi	9	700	7,000	21,000
Bronchi	6	570	5,700	17,100
Bronchi	4	190	1,900	5,700
Bronchi	1	35	350	1,050

*Reprinted with permission from *Physiological Reviews* 41:314, 1961.

Gas density is more important than gas viscosity in conditions of turbulent flow. Advantage of this fact is taken in the utilization of gas mixtures less dense than ordinary room air to reduce problems with airflow resistance. From Table 6-3, it can be seen that helium is about 7 times less dense than nitrogen. A helium-oxygen gas mixture, because of its lower viscosity and total weight, has been recommended for aerospace cabins, although presently 100% oxygen at about one-third atmospheric pressure is utilized. This elevated P_IO_2 (about 250 mmHg) will depress red blood cell production if breathed for extended periods.

THE WORK AND THE OXYGEN COST OF BREATHING

We have already seen that an increase in the resistance to breathing brings with it an increased energy requirement if the breathing rate and depth are to be maintained. Stated another way, when the resistance to breathing is increased, a greater pressure must be created to bring about a given volume of air transfer, which implies that the muscles of ventilation must generate more tension. The system must work harder. The work of breathing is calculated as the product of volume changes (in ml) and applied pressure changes (in gm/cm²). The units of work are gm-cm in this instance (gm/cm² x cm³ ; remember that 1ml = 1cc = 1cm³).

During quiet breathing about 65% of the work done (2,500 gm-cm) overcomes elastic resistance, and 35% (1,400 gm-cm) overcomes viscous or frictional forces. A ventilatory frequency of 12 breaths per minute would represent a work load of 3,900 x 12 = 46,800 gm-cm/min. Ventilatory muscles have an efficiency of about 10%, and the O_2 equivalent of 1,000 gm-cm of work has been estimated as 0.5ml. Using this information, we can estimate the O_2 utilization by the ventilatory muscles at rest as: 46,800 gm-cm/min x 0.10 x 0.5 ml O_2/1,000 gm-cm = 2.3 ml/min. The typical resting O_2 consumption of healthy adults is 250ml/min. thus, only about 0.9% of the total resting O_2 consumption is utilized by the ventilatory muscles.

As ventilation increases, the O_2 needs of ventilatory muscles also rise, somewhat linearly until moderate activity levels, but then increase out of of proportion to the total O_2 uptake. When ventilation reaches about 70 L/min., about 30% of the total O_2 consumption goes to providing ventilation itself. This can increase to as high as 50–75% at maximum exercise. The body is a self-optimizing machine, meeting its ventilatory needs with a combination of breathing rate and depth that keeps elastic and resistance forces minimal.

Unfortunately, in disease states such as advanced pulmonary emphysema, the O_2 cost of ventilation at rest can be 25–30% of the total. The cost of further increases in ventilation, as with exercise, may so far exceed the additional O_2 provided by the increased effort that the ends do not justify the means. For such patients, even a small amount of movement adds greatly to O_2 demands. One solution is to increase the O_2 content of the inspired gas, thereby countering any further reduction in blood O_2 (hypoxemia) and minimizing the acidotic effects of elevated blood CO_2 (hypercapnic acidosis).

RELEVANT READING

Abramovitz, S., Leiner, G.C., Lewis, W.A., et al. Vital capacity in the Negro. *American Review of Respiratory Disease* **92**:287–292, 1965.

Agostoni, E. Mechanics of the pleural space. *Physiological Reviews* **52**:57–128, 1972.

Anonymous. ATS Statement—Snowbird Workshop on Standardization of Spirometry. *American Review of Respiratory Disease* **119**:831–838, 1979.

Bobear, J.B. Obstructive airways disease. *Postgraduate Medicine* **60**(3): 177–185, 1976.

Cosio, M., Ghezzo, H., Hogg, J.C., et al. The relation between structural changes in small airways and pulmonary function tests. *New England Journal of Medicine* **298**:1277–1281, 1978.

Cotes, J.E. *Lung function: Assessment and application in medicine*, 2nd ed. Philadelphia: F.A. Davis, 1979.

Craig, D.B., Wahba, W.M., Don, M.F., Coutre, J.G., and Becklake, M.R. Closing volume and its relationship to gas exchange in seated and supine positions. *Journal of Applied Physiology* **31**:717–721, 1971.

Francis, P.B. Spirometry in office practice. *Postgraduate Medicine* **63**(1):72–81, 1978.

Gaensler, E.A., and Wright, G.W. Evaluation of respiratory impairment. *Archives of Environmental Health* **12**:146–189, 1966.

Hepper, N.G., Black, L.F., and Fowler, W.S. Relationships of lung volume to height and arm span in normal subjects and in patients with spinal deformity. *American Review of Respiratory Disease* **91**:356–362, 1965.

Hogg, J.C., Macklem, P.T., and Thurlbeck, W.M. Site and nature of airway obstruction in chronic obstructive lung disease. *New England Journal of Medicine* **278**:1355–1360, 1968.

Macklem, P.T. Obstruction in small airways: A challenge to medicine. *American Journal of Medicine* **52**:721–724, 1972.

Mead, J. Mechanical properties of the lungs. *Physiological Reviews* **41**:281–330, 1961.

Miller, W.F. Chronic obstructive pulmonary disease. *Hospital Practice* **16**(2):89–106, 1981.

Morris, J.F., Koski, A., and Johnson, L.C. Prediction nomograms (BTPS), spirometric values in normal males and females. *American Review of Respiratory Disease* **103**:57–67, 1971.

Morris, J.F., Temple, W., and Koski, A. Normal values for the ratio of one-second forced expiratory volume to forced vital capacity. *American Review of Respiratory Disease* **108**:1000–1003, 1973.

Oscherwitz, M., Edlavitch, S.A., Baker, T.R., et al. Differences in pulmonary functions in various racial groups. *American Journal of Epidemiology* **96**:319–327, 1972.

Petty, T.L. Spirometry in clinical practice. *Postgraduate Medicine* **69**(4):122–132, 1981.

Ruppel, G. *Manual of pulmonary function testing,* 2nd ed. St. Louis: C.V. Mosby, 1979.

Ward, P.C.J. Pleural fluid data. *Postgraduate Medicine* **72**(4):281–304, 1982.

Weast, R.C., ed. *Handbook of Chemistry and Physics,* 64th ed. Boca Raton: CRC Press, 1983.

Webster, I.W. Spirometry in assessing non-obstructive ventilatory impairment. *Respiration* **31**:97–104, 1974.

Surface Tension Relationships in the Lung

Chapter Seven

Chapter Seven Outline

The chest, because of the arrangement of its distensible elements, tends to expand. Because the lungs are tied to the chest by way of the pleural membranes, they do not collapse unless this functional connection is removed. (This can in fact occur with a pneumothorax). Just as important in explaining the mechanics of respiration are the unique surface properties of a thin fluid layer lining all the alveoli. This specialized fluid, called surfactant, is produced by alveolar Type II cells. Without it, the large surface area within the lungs, so important for ensuring gas exchange with the circulating blood, could not be maintained. This Chapter discusses the mechanisms by which effective surface-tension relationships are maintained in the lung, and the problems that can occur when these relationships are disturbed. Elucidation of these mechanisms has required an impressive interaction of such varied disciplines as physics, biochemistry, pathology, and physiology. The benefits for human health, especially with improvements in neonatal care, have been extraordinary.

HISTORICAL AND PHYSICAL CONCEPTS REGARDING LUNG SURFACE TENSION

Karl von Neergaard, a Zurich physician whose ideas were remarkably ahead of his time, was the first person to grapple effectively with the problem of how lungs spread their inspired air so evenly among the millions of alveoli. He, as well as other scientists during the 1920s, were aware that the elastic fibers distributed throughout the lung tissue were extremely important in contributing to the tendency for the lungs to recoil, or become smaller, as they rested in the intact chest cavity. As von Neergaard pondered over the anatomical interrelationships of the lung, he became even more amazed at the extreme smallness of the alveoli, and how they remain open. It is almost as if the inflated lungs were an emulsion of air in tissue. If one attempted to disperse air in a liquid to this extent, an extraordinary detergent would be required to produce as many bubbles so small. Thinking of how detergents can effectively emulsify fat globules, increasing their surface area for digestion (as we see with bile in the intestine), von Neergaard deduced that indeed the lungs probably also have a kind of surface-tension-lowering detergent lining the alveoli.

Von Neergaard was aware of the physical principles involving surface tension and bubble formation involving air and water. It is appropriate to review these principles here before describing his classic experiments. *Figure 7-1* depicts a water droplet interface with air. Mutual attraction pulls the water molecules at this interface more strongly toward the other innermost water molecules. Thus, the droplet tends to assume a spherical shape. In this configuration there is minimum surface area for the given volume, and thus minimum unbalanced forces. The force required to tear the liquid surface apart is a measure of the surface tension. The measurement units are dynes per cm, i.e., the number of dynes required to produce a one cm linear "tear" in the liquid interface, or, using SI units, millinewtons (mN) per meter where one dyne/cm = 1mN/m.

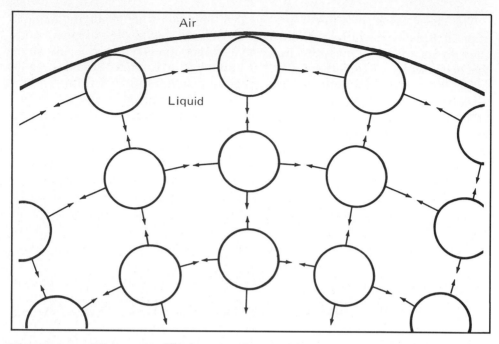

Figure 7-1.   Diagram to illustrate interaction of liquid molecules at an air interface and among themselves within a fluid. Mutual attraction pulls the liquid
molecules at the air interface more strongly toward the other innermost liquid
molecules, and this tends to make the liquid aliquot spherical. *Egan's Fundamentals of Respiratory Therapy* (ed. C.B. Spearman and R.L. Sheldon), p. 135,
C.V. Mosby Co., St. Louis, 1982.

Pierre Simon de LaPlace, a French mathematician, discovered that the surface
tension (T) is related to the pressure (P) inside the droplet and to the droplet's
radius (r) by the relationship: $2T = Pr$ or $P = 2T/r$. In lungs, the situation is slightly
more complex. Instead of water droplets surrounded by air, there are the equivalent of air bubbles (alveoli). Thus there are two surfaces, inner and outer.
LaPlace's mathematical expression for pressure (in Pascals or dyn/cm²) inside
the bubble, of a given radius r (measured in cm) is given by $P = 4T/r$.

We can use an example with real values for the variables involved, and
calculate intra-alveolar pressures when the radius and surface tension values are
known. Let us consider a typical alveolar radius of 200 μm = 0.02cm = 0.0002m.
Assuming that surfactant is present, with a surface tension of about 20 mN/m
= 0.02N/m = 20 dyn/cm, the intra-alveolar pressure can be calculated. Using SI
units, $P = 4T/r = (4 \times 0.020)/0.0002 = 0.08/0.0002 = 400$ Pa = 0.4 kPa = 4 cm
H_2O. Using the CGS system, where 1 kPa = 10,000 dyn/cm² = 10 cm H_2O, P =
$4T/r = (4 \times 20)/0.02 = 4,000$ dyn/cm². Since 1 cm H_2O = 980 gm/cm², then
4,000 dyn/cm² = approximately 4 cm H_2O.

If the surface tension were halved, with the radius remaining unchanged, then the pressure would decrease by a factor of 2. Similarly, if the radius were doubled and the surface tension left unchanged, the pressure would also decrease by a factor of 2. Thus LaPlace's relationship suggests two means for changing the pressure required to keep alveoli open. To reduce the pressure required to keep them open, either the surface tension can be lowered or the radius can be increased.

In the lungs the second alternative is unacceptable. One would not desire all the small alveoli, with their larger pressures, to discharge into neighboring alveoli, with their smaller pressures, to give one huge pulmonary chamber. Ideally, what is desired is the maintenance of large numbers of small alveoli to ensure adequate surface area while still maintaining low surface tension. One does not desire smaller alveoli to merge into larger alveoli.

If there were only a film of water in the alveoli instead of a film of surfactant, water, with its surface tension of 72 mN/m, covering a 0.2 mm alveolus would create, a pressure (P) calculated as $P = 4T/r = (4 \times 0.072)/0.0002 = 1.44$ kPa $= 14.4$ cm H_2O. The adult respiratory musculature is not strong enough to overcome this pressure and inflate the lungs. Thus, insufficient pressure would be created to generate adequate volume changes for ventilation. The lungs would be extremely stiff, or nondistensible. Even if plasma were substituted for water, we would be in a situation similar to the chest-lung system near maximal inflation.

Now we can perhaps understand von Neergaard's experiments and conclusions more easily. He became convinced that surface tension forces contributed to the tendency for the lungs to recoil upon inflation. First, he inflated cat lungs with saline to remove all surface tension effect (Figure 7-2 A). Application of greater and greater inflation pressures brought about nearly linear increases in lung volume. LaPlace's relationship verifies this: the pressure inside a spherical droplet is directly proportional to the droplet surface tension and inversely proportional to the radius of curvature. With saline infusion, and virtually no droplets, essentially no surface tension forces exist, and thus relatively small transpulmonary pressures are needed to maintain any given lung volume. The response of the lung to inflation was very nearly the inverse of deflation.

He inflated the lungs with air. Considerably more pressure was required to produce a volume change equivalent to that with saline filling. Additional pressure was needed to overcome surface tension. Also, the volume/pressure response was different for inflation than for deflation, depicted in Figure 7-2 A. This failure of two reciprocal phenomena to follow similar patterns of response is called *hysteresis*.

Von Neergaard surmised that each alveolus has an air-liquid interface. This liquid is specialized, very different from plasma or saline, and its presence allows the alveoli to retract or recoil just as bubbles do, but also remain open at low inflation pressures. In addition to the elastic connective tissue aspects of lung recoil, the surface material lining the alveolar surfaces also contributes to the hysteresis phenomenon. *Figure 7-2 B* indicates that surface tension forces play a dominant role in lung distensibility at smaller lung volumes, whereas tissue forces (caused primarily by the elastic connective tissue elements) assume increasing importance at larger lung volumes. Nearly 30 years elapsed before the ideas of von Neergaard were fully appreciated.

In 1955 an English toxicologist, R. E. Pattle, revived interest in the need to understand more about this mysterious substance that kept surface tension low on alveolar surfaces. The typical surface tension of water is 72 mN/m, which is so great that small insects can walk on its surface—a pin can float on its surface—without breaking through. The surface tension of mercury is 6.4 times greater (465 mN/m) and that of plasma is intermediate (about 40 mN/m). What is desired in the lungs is a substance that coats the alveoli and which exerts a surface tension certainly no more than that of plasma, preferably much less.

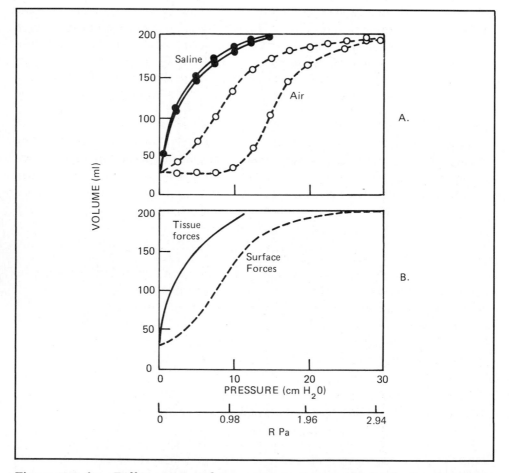

Figure 7-2 A. Difference in volume-pressure curves obtained when lungs are filled with saline and with air. Surface tension forces are almost eliminated with saline filling, hence less pressure is required to produce a given volume. The relative pressure needed to overcome tissue forces and surface tension forces is indicated in 7-2 B. (redrawn with permission from *The Normal Lung*, by J.F. Murray, p. 83, Philadelphia: W.B. Saunders Co., 1976).

Indeed it exists, and in 1957 John Clements provided the first details of its composition. Shortly thereafter this finding was confirmed by other workers. It soon became clear that, while one substance, a lipid named L-dipalmitoyl-lecithin, is present in sizable quantities, the complete secretion of the alveolar Type II cells, called surfactant, is very complex. Not one, but several macromolecules are in this secretion. Their properties change surface tension as alveolar surface area changes. With large lung volumes, the stretched surface film contributes to lung elasticity, but as the lung volumes decrease, compression of the film, with a concomitant reduction in surface tension, tends to prevent alveolar collapse. Thus, by diminishing the recoil force of the lungs at smaller lung volumes, increased stability is provided to a relatively unstable system. The surface tension of lung surface lining material varies from a low of 10 mN/m when the alveoli are at their minimum volume to between 30 and 40 mN/m when they are near their normal expanded state.

Figure 7-3 illustrates an experimental device for investigating surface tension relationships. It is often referred to as a Langmuir-Wilhelmy trough after the two scientists who developed it. The trough is filled with water over which is spread a thin layer of lung surface lining material (surfactant). A movable floating crossbar can vary the thickness of the surfactant layer, which in turn changes the measurable surface tension. For example the surface tension decreases considerably when the crossbar is moved in such a way to concentrate the surfactant mixture. The smaller the surface tension present, the less will be the vertical pull on the platinum strip suspended from a recording gauge.

COMPOSITION AND PRODUCTION OF SURFACTANT

The lipid portion of surfactant is of key importance in lowering surface tension, because of the bipolar nature of its component molecules. The most common and effective molecule in this regard has already been mentioned: L-phosphatidyl-lecithin, also known as dipalmitoyl-lecithin (DPL) or dipalmitoyl-phosphatidylcholine (DPPL). The choline portion of the molecule is hydrophilic or water-attracting; the two saturated fatty acid side chains are hydrophobic, or water-repelling, and lipid-attracting (Figure 7-4). This substance often accounts for more than 50% of the total lipid fraction of surfactant. Lipids produced in lesser quantity include phosphatidylethanolamine, neutral lipids such as cholesterol, acidic phospholipids, and sphingomyelin.

Lowered surface tension throughout the alveolar tissue is a constant requirement in order to reduce the muscular effort required to ventilate the lungs. Thus, surfactant must be continuously secreted, and all alveoli must have the capability of producing it. Each alveolus contains about half a dozen Type II cells. Electron microscopic investigations reveal numerous small membrane-bound vesicles, called inclusion bodies, in each Type II cell. The composition of this

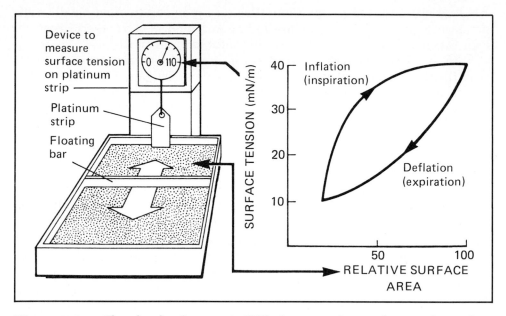

Figure 7-3.   Sketch of a Langmuir-Wilhelmy trough, used to study surface tension forces. Surface tension forces exerted on the platinum strip vary with the area of the film, which can be increased or decreased by moving the floating bar farther from or closer to the platinum strip. (redrawn with permission from *Applied Respiratory Physiology*, by J.F. Nunn, p. 74, Butterworths: Boston, 1977).

vesicle fluid is essentially the same as surfactant. Simple fusion of a vesicle membrane with the Type II cell membrane allows discharge of the vesicle contents onto the alveolar surface. Half of the total amount secreted at any given moment will be metabolized within 14 hours. This short half-life emphasizes the requirement for a high level of metabolic activity in these Type II cells, to ensure continual production.

Normal ventilation is responsible for spreading the layer of surfactant on alveolar surfaces. This is the teleological reason for sighing—it provides a periodic renewal of this material in the under-ventilated alveoli. Thus, mechanical ventilators need to be constructed in such a way that periodic sighing is incorporated into the ongoing breathing rhythm.

Apart from lowering surface tension, surfactant appears to have additional roles. By spreading continuously to areas of lesser surfactant concentration, it moves bacteria, and other small particles, preventing them from settling and increasing the chances for phagocytic alveolar macrophages to encounter and ingest them. It may also prevent transudation of water from the circulatory system during most of a respiratory cycle, reducing the incidence of pulmonary edema. No biologic substance has been discovered that has lower surface tension properties than surfactant.

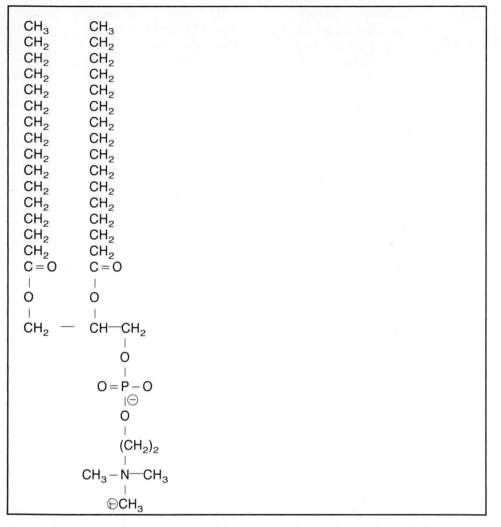

Figure 7-4.   Biochemical structure of dipalmitoyl-phosphatidylcholine. The hydrophobic portion is composed of the palmitic acid moieties, which are insoluble in water. The hydrophilic, or water-attracting portion, is phosphatidyl-choline.

HORMONAL INFLUENCES ON SURFACTANT PRODUCTION

The precise controlling mechanisms that govern production and turnover of surfactant are beginning to be identified. Thyroxine is an important *in vivo* regulator of lipid metabolism, and has been suggested as a possible regulator of surfactant production. Studies with experimental animals that were administered thyroxine have suggested, on the basis of morphological changes in the alveolar Type II cells, an increased storage and production of surfactant. A similar situation has been demonstrated in humans. The frequency and severity of respiratory distress in newborn children has been inversely linked to low umbilical cord thyroid hormone levels. A delay in fetal thyroid gland development may explain the relationship.

Experimental and clinical observations suggest that adrenal glucocorticoid hormones have an important role in the maturation of fetal lung tissue of several species, including man. In both lambs and rabbits, which have been studied extensively, administration of glucocorticoid hormones to the fetus accelerates Type II cell maturation, increases surfactant production and improves pulmonary function.

SURFACTANT AND FETAL DEVELOPMENT

In human fetuses, alveolar Type II cells are first observed about the 26th week of gestational life, and are readily apparent by the 28th to 32nd weeks. These cells begin to produce surfactant in sizable quantities at about the 27th week, as seen by the measurement of lecithin (DPPL) and sphingomyelin in amniotic fluid collected by amniocentesis, a procedure involving the transabdominal aspiration of this fluid by syringe. Lecithin levels rise faster than sphingomyelin, and a ratio of the two (greater than 3.5), referred to as the L/S ratio, was used in early studies to indicate that lung development was proceeding on schedule.

More recently, it has become possible to test the ability for surfactant material, recovered by amniocentesis, to generate a stable surface foam when shaken with 95% ethanol. The saturated fatty acid components (notably DPPL) will form highly stable surface films that can support the structure of a foam for relatively long periods.

A sharp increase in the total amniotic fluid steroid hormone concentration (notably cortisol) begins after the 34th week of gestation. The source of this cortisol is the fetal adrenal glands, and its presence is an important factor in the process of fetal lung maturation. If the fetal adrenal is somewhat slow in its maturation, or if any of several situations prompt premature fetal delivery, one might expect pulmonary complications as a result of inadequate amounts or inappropriate composition of surfactant lining the lungs. The administration of certain corticosteroid medications 12 hours prior to a pre-term delivery can accelerate the maturation process in surfactant-producing lung tissue.

One of the leading causes of premature infant death in the United States is an idiopathic (naturally-occurring) respiratory distress syndrome (IRDS) caused by a deficiency of pulmonary surfactant. The syndrome is characterized by a greatly increased recoil force in the lungs, with a tendency for their collapse. This results in a combination of labored breathing, cyanosis, and a phenomenon called atelectasis (literally, 'incomplete extension,' referring to the regions of the lung which have never become aerated, as opposed to regions that once were aerated but which now are collapsed). The end result is, of course, hypoxia (decreased tissue oxygenation) and acidemia (lowered blood pH).

Many factors can increase the risk of a pregnancy not going completely to term. Among these are repeat Cesarean sections, diabetes, Rh sensitization (erythro-blastosis fetalis), placental insufficiency, pre-eclampsia, and toxemia. An obstetrician is thus faced with the dilemma of either allowing the pregnancy to continue to term with its associated risk of intrauterine death, or terminating the pregnancy and delivering a premature infant who may suffer from IRDS. For this reason, the ability to assess the level of fetal lung development by examining the status of surfactant-producing cells has been welcomed greatly.

Theoretically, with time, the syndrome should be self-limiting. Following delivery, eventual growth and maturation of the surfactant-producing system should permit development of normal lung function. A perplexing problem has been how to maintain the prematurely-born infant, with its tendency toward respiratory failure, in a stable condition until that growth and maturation occurs. The implementation of continuous positive airway pressure (CPAP) ventilation has been very effective for this. To understand how CPAP works, we must apply some additional physiological concepts.

It should be clear already that the lungs are a constantly changing system of alveoli and blood vessels that are alternately opening and closing, or getting larger or smaller, depending on the balance of pressures within these structures (intramural) and outside these structures (interstitial). Alan Burton studied extensively the blood vessels in this regard. In 1951 he coined the term *critical closing pressure* in reference to the tendency for small blood vessels to close because of inherent tension in their walls, even when intramural pressure was greater than interstitial (extravascular) pressure. In alveoli a similar relationship occurs. Surface tension prevents a collapsed alveolus from inflating until a critical opening pressure is reached, at which time it pops open. Then, it can be increased in volume somewhat with even less pressure *(Figure 7-5)*. Further inflation will require additional pressure, and will eventually challenge the elastic limits of the alveolus. This then becomes the limiting factor for its maximum volume. Similarly with deflation, although the volume-pressure rela-tionship is quantitatively different, reflecting the immediately past "history" of its volume change, at a critical closing pressure the alveolus will suddenly close. Surface tension determines volume-pressure relationships primarily when these are small, but as they get larger, tissue elasticity becomes the important determin-ing factor.

The alveoli of premature infants born with IRDS have a different volume-pressure relationship because of their paucity of surfactant. Still, considerable work is required to inflate closed alveoli through and beyond their critical opening pressure. Thus, if these alveoli could be prevented from emptying down to their critical opening volume, they would not quickly close to their resting

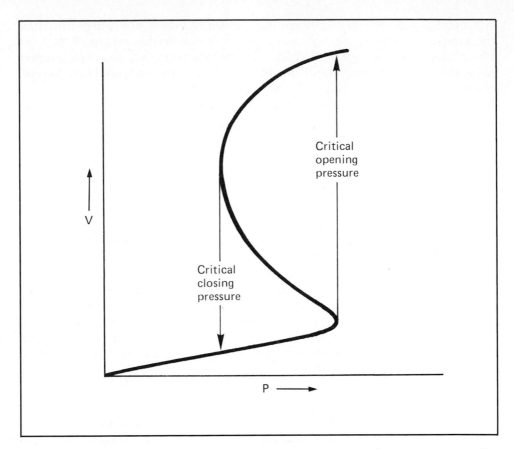

Figure 7-5. As the inflation pressure increases on an alveolus that is essentially deflated, a critical pressure will be reached at which the alveolus very rapidly inflates, and not as much pressure is required to keep it open. The same phenomenon occurs with an inflated alveolus being slowly deflated; here there is a critical pressure for closing the alveolus, or rapidly reducing its volume. (Redrawn with permission from *Respiratory Physiology*, by N.B. Slonim and L.H. Hamilton, 3rd ed., p. 59, The C.V. Mosby Co.: St. Louis, 1976).

volume, and would not require as much pressure to re-open. Continuous positive airway pressure (CPAP) ventilation assists to reduce the work of breathing by maintaining the lung volumes slightly increased. In addition to the concept of critical opening pressure, Laplace's theorem also suggests that CPAP should be of value simply because it keeps the alveoli from closing as much as they ordinarily would. The pressure required to keep an alveolus open could be reduced by half if its radius were doubled.

One synonym for respiratory distress syndrome is *hyaline membrane disease*. This term refers to an additional complication of the syndrome characterized by the presence of a glistening fibrin membrane in the alveolar lining (the Greek word "hyalos" means "glass"). This membrane is derived from the transudation of plasma into the alveoli that can form when insufficient surfactant material is present. Understanding surface tension relationships permits one to see how this membrane might form. Pulmonary surfactant reduces the tendency for water to move from the pulmonary capillaries into the alveoli. Lack of surfactant does the reverse, with alveolar transudation likely.

The problem of inadequate surfactant is not confined to the fetus. In a variety of other situations, such as O_2 toxicity, lung trauma, septicemia, and vascular shock, edema in the lung interstitium and alveoli disrupts normal surface tension relationships. Lung elastic recoil can be increased enormously, with ventilatory assistance mandatory to maintain life in critical situations.

VOLUME-PRESSURE RELATIONSHIPS: COMPLIANCE

We have seen that study of lung volume changes resulting from application of varying external pressure has been useful for understanding the importance of surface tension relationships. Such studies have also provided perspective on the interaction between chest and lungs in permitting inflation to occur with minimal energy cost. Inflation increases both chest and lung volumes. A greater muscular force causes a greater volume change; a greater inspiratory force will bring more lung/chest inflation.

The term *compliance* represents the ease with which lung volume (or chest volume) is changed when a given transpulmonary pressure is applied. It is the slope of the line formed when such volume changes are plotted against transpulmonary changes. *Figure 7-6* illustrates compliance curves for the lung and chest alone, and for the two combined. The more vertical the slope, the greater is the compliance, or ease of increasing volume with increasing inflation pressure.

Compliance implies distensibility or stretchability, which is the opposite of stiffness. Stiffness is somewhat akin to elasticity, defined as the ease with which tissues resist stretch. Elasticity is a measure of the tendency for the lungs to return to their original shape after the application of an inflation pressure.

Compliance is not resistance. Resistance involves a relationship between pressure and flow—kPa per liter per second, or cm H_2O per liter per second—and is measured during motion, not during static conditions. The units of compliance are L/cm H_2O or L/kPa.

To investigate such volume/pressure relationships, two measurement procedures are used. One utilizes body plethysmography (recall *Figure 6-3*) to measure pressure within the lungs at varying volumes when the ventilatory muscles are completely relaxed. Subjects clamp their nose shut, and use mouth breathing to achieve selected well-known lung volume positions, such as FRC, FRC + TV, or TLC. Then they relax their ventilatory muscles, leaving their glottis open, and intra-alveolar pressure is measured at the shutter of the plethysmograph. *Figure*

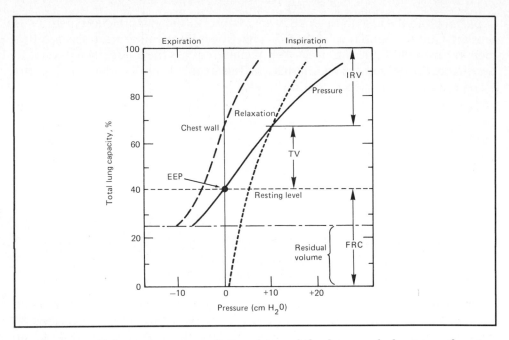

Figure 7-6. Volume-pressure relationships of the lung and chest together (relaxation pressure), and separately. (adapted from Rahn et al., *American Journal of Physiology*. 146:161–178, 1946)

7-6 illustrates the so-called relaxation curve that results when the intraalveolar (or intrapulmonary) pressures at each of the selected lung volumes are graphed.

The other procedure involves the actual estimation of lung compliance itself. The procedure is an indirect one. A nasal tube is inserted and positioned into the lower esophagus. A small balloon at the end is inflated slightly, allowing measurement of the intraesophageal (and thus, intrathoracic, or intrapleural) pressure at various lung volumes. Data from such measurements, when graphed, produce the lung curve in *Figure 7-6*. Using the relaxation and lung curve information, chest compliance can also be determined. This is also indicated in *Figure 7-6*.

First, examine the chest curve. At the EEP, the chest volume is equal to about 70% of the entire lung volume, and thus can accommodate the lungs easily as they inflate during a normal TV. When the lungs inflate very much beyond the normal TV, then the muscles of ventilation must work to enlarge both the chest and lungs together.

The resting end-expiratory position (EEP) is located where the combination curve for both chest and lungs intersects the vertical line drawn through the point indicating zero difference between atmospheric and transpulmonary pressures. Logically, at this position the inward recoil force of the lung is equal and opposite to the outward recoil of the chest wall. The lungs are inflated to FRC, which is about 40% of VC.

Finally, examine the curve for the lungs alone. Its slope is nearly vertical. Thus, there is great ease in inflating the lungs within normal volume limits. The lungs are very distensible, and thus very compliant, thanks in good measure to minimum surface tension forces, but also to stretchable tissues.

An inflation pressure change of 5 cm H_2O (0.5 kPa) will cause a 1L increase in lung volume in adult humans. Thus, the compliance of such lungs is 1L/5 cm H_2O, or 0.2 L/cm H_2O. Using SI units, C_L = 1L/0.5 kPA = 2.0 L/kPa. Realize, of course, that a given inflation pressure will put more air into the lungs of a human than into the lungs of mouse. Thus, compliance decreases with decreasing lung volume. To remove this influence of varying lung volumes, compliance is often expressed in terms of a given unit of lung volume (e.g., L/cm H_2O/L). Clinically, the term *specific compliance* refers to C_L/FRC.

Considerable debate has occurred concerning a possible explanation for the shape of the volume-pressure curve for the lung. Stretching of the elastic fibers may explain the steep lower portion, whereas the flat upper portion relates to the action of collagen fibers as they reach their limits of distensibility. Recent studies of pulmonary emphysema patients have shed light on this idea. These patients have an even steeper lower slope than that observed in healthy lungs, suggesting a disruption of elastic fibers. In 1963 Laurell and Eriksson reported a rare genetic form of pulmonary emphysema, characterized by inadequate circulating quantities of a protease enzyme inhibitor called α_1-antitrypsin. This normally-circulating plasma enzyme prevents destruction of the elastic components of lung tissue by minimizing effects of another normally circulating enzyme, elastase. Emphysematous lungs frequently have sizable destruction of elastic tissue elements.

A fibrotic lung is less compliant than a healthy lung because it is more elastic (stiffer, less stretchable, less distensible). Most restrictive lung diseases are characterized by a decrease in lung compliance. An emphysematic lung is more compliant than a healthy lung because it is less elastic, due to fewer elastic tissue elements. The lungs of an infant with respiratory distress syndrome are less compliant because their reduced quantity of surfactant makes them stiffer.

RELEVANT READING

Brown, E.S., Johnson, R.P., and Clements, J.A. Pulmonary surface tension. *Journal of Applied Physiology* **14:**717–720, 1959.

Burton, A.C. On the physical equilibrium of small blood vessels. *American Journal of Physiology* **164:**319–329, 1951.

Caspi, E., Schreyer, P., and Tamir, I. The amniotic fluid foam test, L/S ratio and total phospholipids in the evaluation of fetal lung maturity. *American Journal of Obstetrics and Gynecology* **122:**323–326, 1975.

Clements, J.A. Surface tension in the lungs. *Scientific American* 207 **(12):** 120–130, 1962.

Clements, J.A. Surface tension of lung extracts. *Proceedings of the Societies for Experimental Biology and Medicine* **95:**170–172, 1957.

Cuestas, R.A., Lindall, A., and Engel, R.R. Low thyroid hormones and respiratory distress syndrome of the newborn. *New England Journal of Medicine* **295:**297–302, 1976.

Finley, T.N., and Ladman, A.J. Low yield of pulmonary surfactant in cigarette smokers. *New England Journal of Medicine* **286:**223–227, 1972.

Hakanson, D.O., and Stern, L. Respiratory distress syndrome of the newborn. *Postgraduate Medicine* 58(3):200–206, 1975.

King, R.J. The surfactant system of the lung. *Federation Proceedings* **33:** 2238–2247, 1974.

Laurell, C.B., and Erikson, S. The electrophoretic α_1-globulin pattern of serum in α_1-antitrypsin deficiency. *Scandinavian Journal of Clinical and Laboratory Investigation* **15:**132–136, 1963.

McDonald, J.E. The shape of raindrops. *Scientific American* 190(2):64–68, 1954.

Morgan, T.E. Pulmonary surfactant. *New England Journal of Medicine* **284:** 1185–1193, 1971.

Pattle, R.E. Properties, function, and origin of the alveolar lining fluid. *Nature* **175:**1125–1126, 1955.

Rahn, H., Otis, A.B., Chadwick, L.E., and Fenn, W.D. The pressure-volume diagram of the thorax and lung. *American Journal of Physiology* **146:**161–178, 1946.

Robert, M.F., Neff, R.K., Hubell, J.P., Taeusch, M.W., and Avery, M.E. Association between maternal diabetes and the respiratory distress syndrome in the newborn. *New England Journal of Medicine* **294:**357–360, 1976.

Pulmonary Gas Exchange

Chapter Eight

Chapter Eight Outline

Gradient Partitioning in the Normal Respiratory System

Diffusion: The Link Between Ventilation and Perfusion

    A. Physical Principles Explaining Diffusion

    B. Linking of Gas Transfer in the Body by Diffusion

    C. Pulmonary Diffusing Capacity

Ventilation

    A. Terminology for Airflow Patterns in Ventilation

    B. Deadspace Ventilation

    C. Non-Uniform Ventilation

Perfusion

    A. Physiology of the Pulmonary Circulation

    B. Concept of Shunt

    C. Non-Uniform Perfusion

Ventilation/Perfusion Ratios and Inequalities

The preceding chapters have described the route taken by environmental gas as it moves from nose and mouth into the lungs. These anatomical considerations have described how this air is cleaned, warmed, and humidified. The ultimate functional unit linking the pulmonary and cardiovascular systems—the alveolo-capillary membrane—has also been identified. The dynamics of achieving appropriate concentrations of the major respiratory gases in the pulmonary capillary blood—O_2 and CO_2—form the logical next step in developing a useful understanding of pulmonary physiology.

The fundamental concepts underlying pulmonary gas exchange are quite simple; application of these principles allows an effective understanding of many disease and dysfunction mechanisms. One concept involves gas flow *gradients*. The body is continually using O_2 and producing CO_2. The partial pressure of the O_2 dissolved in tissues is lower than in atmospheric air; that of CO_2 is higher. These gases thus tend to move in a direction down their concentration gradients, i.e., from regions of higher to lower concentrations. A second concept emphasizes the mechanism by which these gradients allow gas flow, namely *diffusion*. Third, is the crucial concept of *uneven ventilation* of the lung, with its effects on gas exchange with the pulmonary blood. Fourth, is the circulatory equivalent of *uneven perfusion* of blood through the lung, which also reduces efficiency of gas exchange. A general understanding of these concepts will permit consideration of ventilation/perfusion relationships in a knowledgeable manner.

GRADIENT PARTITIONING IN THE NORMAL RESPIRATORY SYSTEM

Breathing allows the exchange of respiratory gases between the external environment and the bloodstream. Of crucial importance is the adequacy of this ventilatory steady state to supply the body's metabolic needs. Gases move from atmosphere to alveoli, and eventually to other tissues, as a result of the concentration differences between these sites. The primary gases involved in metabolism are O_2 and CO_2 although nitrogen comprises the greatest percentage of the total gas exchanged.

The law of John Dalton, an English chemist and physicist, governs such movement by the following relationship: $P_G = F_G \times P_B$, where P_G = the pressure of one of the gases, P_B = barometric (total) pressure, and F_G = the fraction of the total volume which any single gas occupies. As an example, if O_2 represents 20.9% of atmospheric air, then at a barometric pressure of 760 mmHg (101.6 kPa), $PO_2 = 0.209 \times 760 = 158.8$ mmHg (21.2 kPa). Dalton's law implies that each gas can be considered separately and that the sum of the individual gas partial pressures equals the total gas pressure without any special chemical interaction.

Physicists and chemists are often interested in the number of molecules of a gas rather than the volume they occupy. They find it convenient to use as a frame of reference a standard set of conditions: sea level barometric pressure of 760 mmHg (101.3 kPa), 0°C, and with no influence of water vapor on P_B. These conditions are summarily referred to as STPD (Standard Temperature and Pressure, Dry). Our own ambient environment is almost never in this state, because weather fluctuations constantly alter the P_B, the ambient temperature, and the absolute humidity. Table 8-1 compares the partial pressures of the gases involved in breathing in several different environments: 1) under standard dry conditions (0°C, sea-level), 2) typical atmospheric conditions with some humidity, 3) completely humidified conditions at body temperature (such as in the trachea), 4) in the alveoli, and 5) in air just expired from the lungs.

Although P_B is the same in each situation, sizable differences occur in the relative percentage of each gas in the different environments.

Physiologists have another set of conditions that interest them in addition to STPD, namely, BTPS—those conditions in the alveoli. BTPS refers to body temperature, ambient atmospheric pressure, and air saturated with water vapor. P_{H_2O} depends upon temperature and not upon pressure. Usually in the trachea, as well as everywhere below this level in the airway, there is complete humidification of air and warming to body temperature. According to elementary physics principles, the molecules of a liquid, like those of a gas, are in constant motion. Those at the surface tend to escape into the gas above the liquid. The greater the temperature, the greater is the kinetic energy of the molecules, and the greater their tendency to escape. Water vapor at body temperature maintains a partial pressure of 47 mmHg (6.3 kPa) regardless of P_B changes (Table 4-1).

Under resting healthy conditions in a normal environment, flow gradients for O_2 and CO_2 similar to those illustrated in Figure 8-1 are operant. There is a steadily decreasing O_2 availability from ambient environment (P_IO_2) to trachea ($P_{trach}O_2$) to alveolus (P_AO_2) to arterial blood (P_aO_2) to interstitial fluid ($P_{ISF}O_2$) to metabolizing cell ($P_{cell}O_2$) and finally to mitochondria ($P_{mito}O_2$). This is sometimes referred to as the O_2 cascade. A similar increase in PCO_2 occurs in the opposite direction, from the cell to the alveolus. However, P_aCO_2 is greater than ($P_{trach}O_2$), which in turn is greater than P_ECO_2, because of dilution with environmental air.

Equilibrium between alveolar and lung capillary blood O_2 and CO_2 occurs very rapidly. The $P_{\bar{v}}O_2$ of 40 mmHg (5.3 kPa) rises to virtual equilibration with P_AO_2, at 100 mmHg (13.3 kPa). Similarly, the $P_{\bar{v}}CO_2$ of 46 mmHg (6.1 kPa) falls such that P_ACO_2 ends up at 40 mmHg (5.3 kPa). Normally, there is only about 0.75 sec available for these exchanges, but equilibration is complete within half that time. This provides an enormous margin of safety for exercise.

Three concepts of considerable significance should be made clear at this point. One is that the P_AO_2 and P_ACO_2 are not the same as the $P_{\bar{E}}O_2$ and $P_{\bar{E}}CO_2$ (i.e., the mean expired gas partial pressures). Also, the $P_{LC}O_2$ and $P_{LC}CO_2$ (where LC = lung capillary) are not the same as the P_aO_2 and P_aCO_2 found in blood exiting the heart or in the pulmonary vein draining the lungs. The reason for this is that not always are all well-perfused pulmonary capillaries in intimate contact with well-ventilated alveoli. We will describe this apparent ventilation/perfu-

TABLE 8-1. Partial Pressures of Respiratory Gases Under Different Environmental Conditions

GAS	Dry conditions 0°C; sea-level			Moist Air Some humidity			Tracheal Gas; 37°C 100% Humidity			Alveolar Gas 100% Humidity			Expired Gas 100% Humidity		
	mm Hg	kPa	%	mm Hg	kPa	%	mm Hg	kPa	%	mm Hg	kPa	%	mm Hg	kPa	%
N_2	600.6	80.1	79.03	597.0	79.5	78.62	563.4	75.1	74.09	569.0	75.8	74.90	566.0	75.4	74.50
O_2	159.1	21.2	20.93	159.0	21.2	20.84	149.3	19.9	19.67	104.0	13.9	13.60	120.0	16.0	15.70
CO_2	0.3	0.04	0.04	0.3	0.04	0.04	0.3	0.04	0.04	40.0	5.3	5.30	27.0	3.6	3.60
H_2O	0.0	0.0	0.00	3.7	0.5	0.50	47.0	6.3	6.20	47.0	6.3	6.20	47.0	6.3	6.20
TOTAL	760.0	101.3	100.00	760.0	101.3	100.00	760.0	101.3	100.00	760.0	101.3	100.00	760.0	101.3	100.00

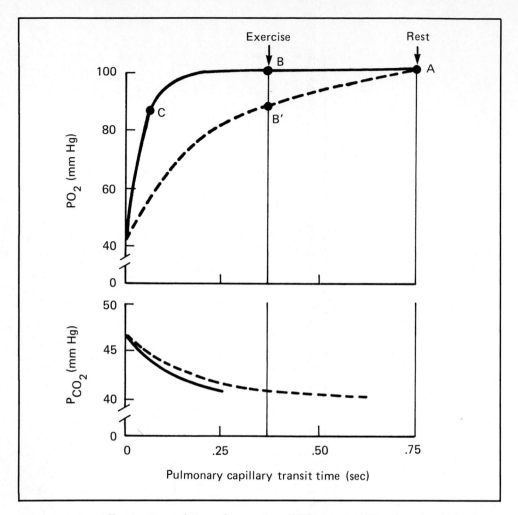

Figure 8-1.   Illustration of time dynamics of PO_2 and PCO_2 changes in pulmonary capillaries under various conditions. The solid lines represent conditions
with normal alveolocapillary membranes: under resting conditions (A) complete equilibration occurs, and even with exercise (B) this happens. The dashed
lines represent the effect of decreased diffusing capacity, for example, with a
thickened alveolocapillary membrane. Greater time is required for equilibratium
of both gases, but for O_2 the effect is worse due to its lesser solubility. (Reprinted
with permission from *The Normal Lung*, by J. F. Murray, p. 177, W. B. Saunders
Co., Philadelphia, 1976.)

sion mismatch in greater detail later in this chapter. It is important at this
juncture to realize that virtually complete equilibration will occur between any
given alveolus and pulmonary capillary with respect to O_2 and CO_2 whenever
the two structures are in close contact.

The second concept is that a greater volume of O_2 is taken up by the blood than the volume of CO_2 removed from it into the alveolar gas, except during vigorous exercise. This implies that the inspired tidal volume (V_I) will be larger than the expired tidal volume (V_E). Nitrogen is not one of the gases exchanged at the alveolocapillary membrane. Thus, the expired N_2 (F_EN_2) will be greater than the inspired N_2 (F_IN_2) by an amount just equal to the difference between CO_2 release and O_2 uptake. Thus, $\dot{V}_I = \dot{V}_E \times (F_EN_2/F_IN_2)$.

The third concept is that respiratory gases move across the alveolocapillary membrane by diffusion alone, and not by any active secretory process. This question plagued the minds of some of the best scientists for 30 years. In the 1890s the famous Danish physiologist Christian Bohr had become convinced that under certain stressful conditions, such as exercise at high altitude, diffusion alone was inadequate. In 1909, he published a classic paper summarizing 20 years of research on the subject. It was one of his most famous students, August Krogh (together with Marie Krogh, his wife), who disagreed and developed the necessary technology to state confidently in 1910 that the partial pressure of O_2 in alveolar gas was always greater than that in arterial blood (i.e., $P_AO_2 > P_aO_2$).

Two years later, a paper published by Charles Douglas, John Scott Haldane and their colleagues, following a expedition to Pikes Peak in Colorado (14,100 ft., 4,300 m) produced data to the contrary. Once again, P_aO_2 was greater than P_AO_2 by as much as 35 mmHg (4.7 kPa). Thus, some kind of active transport (secretory) had to occur. The debate was put to rest finally by Joseph Barcroft who in 1920 lived in a glass chamber for six days, under simulated conditions of hypoxia and exercise. Essentially, he duplicated the Pikes Peak experiments in his own laboratory, allowing blood collection from his surgically exposed radial artery. There was little doubt that secretion did not in fact occur, and that the previous confusion related to methodological problems in data collection.

Barcroft wrote three most fascinating books, each with the same title: *The Respiratory Function of the Blood,* in which he lucidly explained the concepts then known about respiratory physiology. He had become an intimately personal expert in the problems of O_2 diffusion, realizing full well that, were it not for the extraordinary surface area of the lungs, indeed some process other than mere diffusion would be required. Writing in his first book, he put it this way: except for the existence of hemoglobin, "man might never have attained any activity which the lobster does not possess, or had he done so, it would have been with a body as minute as the fly's."

DIFFUSION: THE LINK BETWEEN VENTILATION AND PERFUSION

A. PHYSICAL PRINCIPLES EXPLAINING DIFFUSION

Diffusion is the physical process by which gas molecules move from a region of greater concentration to one of lesser concentration. Such migration is secondary to the Brownian movement of particles. Although movement continues when concentrations of the gas are equal in both regions, no net movement (change in concentration) occurs, and an equilibrium exists. Two factors determine how rapidly gases will move across the alveolocapillary membrane. One is the molecular weight, the other is solubility. Two physical principles describe the relationship more fully.

The law of Thomas Graham deals with diffusion of gases in an all-gas phase as well as with their movement through both gas and liquid phases. The latter is relevant for our consideration of gases diffusing from alveoli into blood. Graham realized that the diffusion of gas into a liquid is directly proportional to its solubility coefficient (designated by the Greek letter alpha), and indirectly proportional to the square root of its molecular weight or density.

The molecular weight of O_2 is 32, that of CO_2 is 44. Thus, if solubility were not a factor (which would be true in an all-gas phase), O_2 should diffuse through the gas mixture slightly faster ($\sqrt{44}/\sqrt{32} = 6.63/5.66 = 1.17$ times) than CO_2. For gases to dissolve in fluids, however, solubility becomes an important variable. The solubility coefficient (α) is defined as the volume of gas (STPD) in ml which will dissolve in one ml of fluid (here, plasma). The α for O_2 is 0.023 ml/ml at 38°C; for CO_2 it is 0.510. Thus, from solely the viewpoint of solubility, CO_2 should have a much greater tendency than O_2 to diffuse into plasma (0.510/0.023 = 22.2 times greater). When the effect of both solubility and molecular weight are considered together, CO_2 is still about 19 times greater in its dissolvability into plasma, as seen by the following calculations:

$$\text{Ratio} = \frac{\alpha\ CO_2 \times \sqrt{O_2\ MW}}{\alpha\ O_2 \times \sqrt{CO_2\ MW}} = \frac{0.510 \times \sqrt{32}}{0.023 \times \sqrt{44}} = \frac{0.510 \times 5.66}{0.023 \times 6.63} = \frac{2.89}{0.152} = 19$$

The principle of William Henry allows quantification of the gas (C_G) that will dissolve in a liquid, through consideration of the solubility of the gas and its partial pressure. Typically, the content (C) of dissolved gas (G) is expressed as ml of that gas per 100 ml of solution (volumes percent). Thus,

$$C_G = \frac{\alpha_G \times 100 \times P_G(mmHg)}{760} = \frac{\alpha_G \times 100 \times P_G\ (kPa)}{101.3}$$

As an example, typically $P_aO_2 = 100$ mmHg (101.3 kPa). Thus, arterial blood O_2 content is calculated as

$$C_aO_2 = \frac{\alpha O_2 \times 100 \times P_aO_2}{760} = \frac{0.023 \times 100}{760} \times 100 = 0.003 \times 100 = 0.3\ \text{Vol\%.}$$

Or, using SI units,

$$C_aO_2 = \frac{\alpha O_2 \times 100 \times P_aO_2}{101.3} = \frac{0.023 \times 100}{101.3} \times 13.3 = 0.023 \times 13.3 = 0.3\ \text{Vol \%.}$$

For ease in remembering how to calculate dissolved O_2 when PO_2 is known, it is thus a simple matter to multiply PO_2 by 0.003 (or 0.023 in SI units.) With CO_2 having a solubility coefficient in plasma of 0.510, the appropriate constant is given by $\alpha CO_2 \times 100/760 = 0.510 \times 100/760 = 0.067$ (or in SI units, 0.510 × 100/101.3 = 0.50). Thus, with P_aCO_2 equal to 40 mmHg (5.3 kPa), $C_a CO_2$ is given by 0.067 × 40 (or 0.50 × 5.3), or 2.7 vol %.

Henry's law describes a linear relationship between gas partial pressure and the amount of gas dissolved. As an example, PO_2 values of 1 mmHg (0.133 kPa), 100 mmHg (13.3 kPa) and 1,000 mmHg (133 kPa) will allow dissolution of 0.3, 0.03, and 3 ml O_2/100 ml blood, respectively.

We have thus described O_2 and CO_2 from the standpoint of four methods of quantification:

1. PARTIAL PRESSURE, the pressure or driving force to move within the gas phase. For O_2, $P_IO_2 = 159$ mmHg (21.1 kPa).
2. TENSION, the tendency to dissolve in the liquid phase. For O_2, the $P_aO_2 = 100$ mmHg.
3. PERCENT COMPOSITION, represented by the relative proportion of gas to the entire gas mixture. For O_2, $F_IO_2 = 0.21$ (21%).
4. DISSOLVED CONTENT, represented by the number of ml of gas per unit (100 ml) of blood, sometimes termed volumes percent. For O_2, $C_aO_2 = 0.30$ vol %.

Because O_2 and CO_2 can bind chemically to several molecules in blood, such as plasma proteins and hemoglobin, there is a fifth aspect of quantification, namely *bound content* of gas. Whereas typically about 0.3 ml O_2 and 3.3 ml CO_2 are dissolved per 100 ml of arterial blood, the chemically bound forms of O_2 and CO_2 are present in much greater quantity, about 20 ml and 50 ml/100 ml, respectively. The details explaining this enormous volume of gas transport in the bound form will be considered in Chapter Nine.

B. LINKING OF GAS TRANSFER IN THE BODY BY DIFFUSION

From a pulmonary point of view, the diffusion link between alveolus and capillary membrane is the essence of gas exchange. However, the ultimate intent of breathing is to provide living tissues, particularly their mitochondria, with sufficient O_2 to permit complete fuel metabolism. CO_2 removal, of course, is also important, but were it not for the O_2 delivery, the CO_2 would not be produced. Thus, there are several other diffusion links that are operative in this chain of events connecting the outside environment to each cell. *Figure 8-2* illustrates these, and emphasizes the inseparable interaction of the cardiovascular and pulmonary systems.

It should be clear by now that not all gases diffuse into the body with equal swiftness, as has been mentioned. Some have limitations placed upon them which are more diffusion-oriented, whereas others are more perfusion-limited in their movement. The best example of diffusion-limited gas transfer is that of carbon monoxide (CO), and because of this it is often used in studying the diffusion capability of the lungs. Blood has an enormous capacity for CO, since hemoglobin's affinity for it is 200–250-fold greater than that for oxygen. As fast as CO can diffuse into the blood it will be bound to hemoglobin.

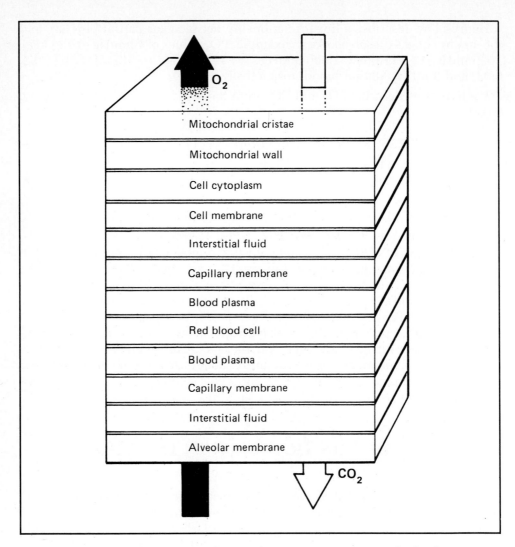

Figure 8-2. The diffusion pathway of respiratory gases in the body.

Oxygen is somewhere in between this extreme and that of nitrous oxide (N_2O), a perfusion-limited gas. Because of the low solubility of N_2O in blood, not much enters unless lung perfusion is quite substantial. Oxygen has greater solubility than N_2O and in addition can bind to hemoglobin, though not as quickly as CO.

Several factors must be considered in assessing the extent to which the optimum quantity of arterial O_2, dissolved in the fluid portion of blood and bound to hemoglobin, can be maintained in the bloodstream. One is the inspired PO_2— the amount of O_2 available for breathing. Another is the amount of O_2 remaining in the mixed venous blood after systemic circulation is complete—this indicates how much O_2 was used, and what the ongoing metabolic needs may have been. A third is the extent to which ventilation and perfusion match in the lungs. A fourth factor is the pulmonary diffusing capacity—the ability for gases in the lungs to exchange with blood. Each of these factors will be discussed in subsequent sections.

C. PULMONARY DIFFUSING CAPACITY

The pulmonary diffusing capacity (D_L) is the volume of gas (V_G) that can diffuse across the alveolocapillary membranes per unit of time in response to the mean pressure difference existing between alveolar air ($P_{\bar{A}}G$) and capillary blood ($P_{\bar{C}}G$). Thus D_L is the net rate of gas transfer per partial pressure gradient. Typical units would be ml/min/mmHg in the CGS system, or, in the SI system, ml/min/kPa or ml/sec/kPa. There are a variety of physical factors that also must be considered, which generally are lumped together into a constant, D. Thus $V_G = D (P_{\bar{A}}G - P_{\bar{C}}G)$, where D is directly related to the solubility coefficient of the gas (α) and the total surface area (A) available for diffusion, but inversely related to the length (l) of the diffusion pathway and to the square root of the molecular weight. Thus, $D = \alpha Al\sqrt{G_{MW}}$.

The diffusing capacity provides a measure of how easily alveolar O_2 exchanges across the alveolocapillary membrane to reach the hemoglobin molecules within adjacent erythrocytes. Thus, there is a membrane component, relating to surface area, thickness, and physiochemical properties of the alveolocapillary membrane, and as well a perfusion component, relating to capillary blood volume and hematocrit. The surface area available for this physiologic exchange can become enlarged by:

1. increasing the number of pulmonary capillaries with an active circulation,
2. dilating the capillaries already functioning, and
3. increasing the surface area of functioning alveoli.

As an example, exercise does this: the diffusing capacity of an exercising lung is greater than that of the same lung at rest. Trained distance runners typically exhibit increased diffusing capacities because one of their training adaptations is an increased volume of plasma along with an increased red blood cell mass.

Disease states, however, can thicken the alveolocapillary membrane, and lower the diffusing capacity. The typical diffusion pathway through the surface film, alveolar cell, interstitial tissue, and capillary cell, is 0.5μm to 1.5 μm thick. Collagen fibers can enlarge the interstitial space. Pulmonary edema fluid can impede diffusion in two ways: by expanding the interstitial space to cause alveolocapillary block, and by welling into the alveoli and bronchioles to cause airway obstruction.

Oxygen is not necessarily the best gas to study for the measurement of pulmonary diffusing capacity. Indeed, it can combine with hemoglobin with such ease that a large flow gradient should exist. However, carbon monoxide is even more advantageous because of its much more rapid binding, leaving the $P_C CO$ so small that it is negligible. Since O_2 transfer is of greatest interest to us, however, the diffusing capacity value of the lung for carbon monoxide (D_LCO) is appropriately converted into an equivalent for O_2. By use of Graham's and Henry's laws, it can be shown that $D_LCO \times 1.23 = D_LO_2$.

A simple ten-second breath-holding test with a low CO content (0.3%) is often used to measure D_L, starting at the residual volume level. The alveolar air CO content is measured before and after the breathing maneuver. If a normal D_LCO is 30 ml/min/mmHg (225 ml/min/kPa), then $30 \times 1.23 = 37$ ml/min/mmHg or 278 ml/min/kPa for D_LO_2.

There are several physiologic variables that affect the assessment of lung diffusing capacity. First, there is species variability. Humans have 85% to 95% of their alveolar surface covered by pulmonary capillaries. Second, aging decreases D_L resulting from the accompanying loss of internal lung surface area, loss of some pulmonary capillaries, and lowered cardiac index (liters of cardiac output per minute per square meter of body surface area). Third, body surface area must be considered, explainable probably by differences in lung volume and body metabolism. There is an approximately 18 ml/min/mmHg or 135 ml/min/kPa rise in D_L per square meter increase in body surface area.

Fourth, body position changes can significantly alter D_L. An expanded pulmonary capillary bed causes a 14% to 20% rise in D_LCO when a subject moves from the supine to the sitting posture. Fifth, exercise, with its accompanying increase in metabolic rate, can produce a doubling of the resting D_LCO, a finding which is not too surprising when one considers that in hard work cardiac output can rise 5 to 6 times, pulmonary arterial pressures and pulmonary blood volume can double, alveolar ventilation can increase 20 to 30 times, and the overall distribution of pulmonary ventilation to perfusion becomes much more uniform throughout the lung.

Diffusion measurements have considerable clinical significance. D_L is decreased in pulmonary emphysema patients, for example, because of their reduced surface area for gas exchange caused by destruction of alveolar and capillary walls. The D_L also decreases when the total surface area of capillaries is reduced, as with lesions of the lung or in abnormalities of arterial flow to parts of the lung. Disease states involving a thickening and/or separation of the alveolo-capillary membrane also decrease D_L. Examples of this kind of interstitial or alveolar pulmonary fibrosis include poisoning by beryllium or asbestos inhalation, and connective tissue proliferation diseases (such as sarcoidosis, and scleroderma).

A measurement of D_L is a more sensitive indicator of a decrease in O_2 transfer by the lung than simply a measurement of P_aO_2 or arterial O_2 content. If one does discover a decreased D_L, however, one will not know if this is caused by a lengthened diffusion pathway or by a decreased surface area available for diffusion. Sizeable decreases in D_L may occur, however, before blood leaving the alveolar capillaries begins to lose its full oxygenation. So great is the reserve of the O_2 transfer mechanism that the D_LCO can decrease by 25% to 40% before such compromise occurs.

VENTILATION

A. TERMINOLOGY FOR AIRFLOW PATTERNS IN VENTILATION

Normal spontaneous easy breathing is termed *eupnea*. Ventilation satisfies metabolic needs, but as shall soon be pointed out, during normal ventilation the lungs are by no means uniformly ventilated. A ventilatory rate of 12 breaths per minute, with 500 ml per breath, would give an expired minute volume ($\dot{V}_E$) of 6,000 ml.

A pattern of ventilation whereby breathing is difficult or labored, as a result of disease, is called *dyspnea*. If this occurs while recumbent, the term *orthopnea* is frequently used (and it is more representative of cardiac rather than respiratory disease).

When the ventilatory rate is faster than normal, with the depth not necessarily deeper, this is known as *tachypnea*. Many animals use a form of tachypnea called panting for thermoregulation. It may exceed metabolic needs in terms of gas exchange, depending upon its intensity.

Hyperpnea represents an increased rate and depth of ventilation, sufficient to satisfy metabolic needs. Joggers out on an easy afternoon training run would demonstrate exercise hyperpnea. Since resting P_aO_2 and P_aCO_2 values are maintained, their condition could more specifically be called a normoxic isocapnic hyperpnea.

When the ventilatory rate and depth are both increased, but with ventilation in excess of metabolic needs, then *hyperventilation* is occurring. There will be a decreased P_aCO_2 and an increased P_aO_2, the former being much larger and more significant than the latter. A respiratory alkalosis occurs from the loss of CO_2. Hyperventilation can reduce the P_ACO_2 from 40 mmHg to 20 mmHg (5.3 to 2.7 kPa). There is a slight increase in P_AO_2 but this does not substantially increase arterial blood O_2 saturation. This is simply because the system's efficiency normally allows about 97% saturation of the blood with O_2, and any greater increase in P_AO_2 increases the saturation only about 2%.

There are many causes of hyperventilation. Some are nervous in origin: anxiety reactions, extreme pain, and central nervous system lesions stimulate the brain ventilatory centers. Various hormones and drugs, such as epinephrine and salicylates, increase the breathing rate. Increased metabolism from fever or hyperthyroidism, metabolic acidosis from diabetes or kidney problems both elevate blood H^+ concentration, which also stimulates the brain ventilatory centers. Mechanical overventilation from excessive pressure on rebreathing bags or improperly adjusted mechanical ventilators can elicit hyperventilation.

Hypoventilation implies a decreased breathing rate and depth; the individual is simply breathing insufficient air for adequate gas exchange. Not only does the P_aO_2 decrease (hypoxemia), but the P_aCO_2 rises (hypercapnia) as well as the P_ACO_2. Respiratory acidosis is the eventual result. Because CO_2 cannot be eliminated properly, from a physiologic viewpoint hypoventilation is a far more serious consequence than hyperventilation.

It also can occur for many reasons. The brain respiratory centers may be depressed by general anesthesia, morphine, barbiturate overdose, or electrocution. Diseases that adversely affect the ventilatory muscles impair breathing. So does interference with neural conduction or neuromuscular transmission caused by such varied situations as spinal cord injury and neuromuscular block from curare, nerve gases, botulinum toxin, nicotine, and succinylcholine. Pleural effusion or pneumothorax can limit lung movement, thereby inducing hypoventilation.

B. DEAD SPACE VENTILATION

Fish have a one-way flow of gas-containing fluid (fresh or salt water) that passes the circulatory system in their gills. Mammals and birds have a two-way flow of gas, moving from mouth or nose to lungs and back again. In fish, all of the fluid entering the mouth eventually passes the gills and contacts the circulation. In mammals and birds, with alveolocapillary interrelationships only in the innermost portion of the two-way system, a sizeable portion of the gas entering the system never gets to this region of intimate exchange. Functionally, it is ineffective for actual circulatory system exchange, and it is termed *dead space.*

The knowledge that dead space existed has been around since before the turn of the century. Nathan Zuntz made a plaster cast of the respiratory tract in 1882, and eventually it became clear that only after one reaches what Ewald Weibel later termed the 17th generation of divisions of the tracheobronchial tree does one find alveoli. Thus, the *anatomic dead space* is the entire region from upper respiratory tract (nose, mouth, pharynx, etc. which comprises about half the total tract volume) to deep within the lungs where gas exchange with blood still has not begun to occur. Only when respiratory bronchioles are reached, with their occasional alveoli, do we find the beginnings of gas exchange.

Actual estimation of the volume of this anatomic dead space has been an enormous challenge. Many techniques have been employed, each with its own variability, and in addition, a large number of factors can cause it to change. Quite obviously, it should vary depending upon where one is in the ventilatory cycle. Inspiration increases the airway diameters. An open lower jaw will give more volume. Anatomic dead space increases directly and linearly with increasing body height. Administration of bronchodilator or bronchoconstrictor drugs typically increase or decrease dead space, respectively, by virtue of their effects on small airway patency. The anatomic dead space (in ml) in healthy adults at the FRC position is often estimated as the ideal body weight in pounds (i.e., a 160 pound person's anatomic dead space would be 160 ml). This value approximates the value of 162 ml estimated in the detailed studies by Fritz Rohrer published in 1915 and 1916 considering individuals of this same size.

If a tidal volume of 500 ml is inspired, and if the anatomic dead space is 150 ml, then 350 ml consists of ambient air. Assuming that the latter component of the inspired volume ventilates spaces that are well-perfused, then $350/500 \times 100 = 70\%$ of the inspired volume is functional (it participates in gas exchange). On exhalation, the first gas expelled is from the anatomic dead space and is identical in composition to room air. Soon afterwards, some alveolar air will begin to exit, having come from those alveoli closest to the carina (about 17 cm away). As exhalation continues, the alveolar contribution increases, from contribution of the more distant alveoli (up to 40 cm from the carina). Eventually, the last 150 ml will be expelled, which is almost solely alveolar air (it is so high in CO_2 that it will extinguish a candle). The virtually identical CO_2 composition of this final 150 ml among healthy people was first reported in 1905 by John Haldane and John Priestley.

It was Christian Bohr in 1891 who first accurately described the ideas of dead space and alveolar gas composition. Since atmospheric CO_2 is negligible, it must arise in the lungs from metabolism. Thus, alveolar CO_2 concentration ($F_A CO_2$) equals the mixed expired CO_2 concentration ($F_{\overline{E}} CO_2$). Alveolar ventilation is represented by tidal volume (V_T) minus dead space volume (V_D)—it is physiologically usable ventilation. Thus, for each single breath, $F_A CO_2 \times (V_T - V_D) = F_{\overline{E}} CO_2 \times V_T$. Nowadays, is is convenient to use these same principles to estimate the dead space by knowing $F_A CO_2$, $F_{\overline{E}} CO_2$, and V_T. Using data from Table 8-1, the equation is $V_D/V_T = (F_A CO_2 - F_{\overline{E}} CO_2)/F_A CO_2 = 0.053 - 0.036/0.053 = 0.017/0.053 = 0.32$. Thus, about one third of each tidal volume is dead space.

However, in certain pathological situations, there can be considerable dead space in the alveolar region because many capillaries will not be fully functional (Figure 8-3). The best term for this is *alveolar dead space*. It normally adds ten percent to the total dead space ventilation. Thus, $V_D = V_D(ANAT) + V_D(ALV) = 150 \text{ ml} + 15 \text{ ml} = 165 \text{ ml}$, and $V_D/V_T = 165/500 = 0.33$. Alveolar ventilation still equals tidal volume minus dead space volume, or $V_A = V_T - V_D$. The dead space volume, however, can have both anatomic (non-alveolar) and pathophysiologic (alveolar) components.

The explanation for the pathophysiologic dead space is simply one of ineffective pulmonary perfusion—gas delivery is achieved but exchange with blood does not occur. Several examples can illustrate this perfusion problem. One is pulmonary thromboembolism, resulting from migrating clots from lower limbs with thrombophlebitis or fat emboli following the fracture of a bone such as the femur or pelvis. These patients may have shortness of breath, chest pain, cough, and possibly hemoptysis (bronchial or pulmonary hemorrhage, seen as a frothy pink sputum). Cyanosis, tachycardia, and profuse sweating may also occur. Arterial blood gas analysis may reveal low arterial PO_2 but no CO_2 retention. Diffusing capacity is reduced because of the areas with acceptable ventilation but no perfusion.

Another cause of alveolar dead space is hypotension from decreased cardiac output and hemorrhage. A redistribution of blood flow and volume favors the

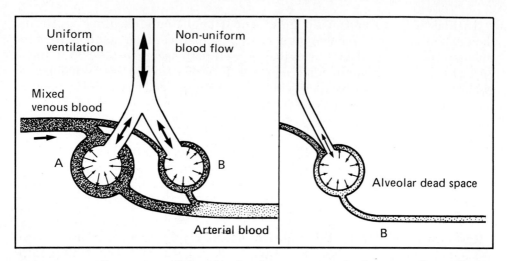

Figure 8-3.   Illustration of alveolar dead space, caused when not all capillaries are fully functional. Ventilation is adequate in alveoli A and B, but the poor perfusion around alveolus B decreases the functional effectiveness of these alveoli for blood gas exchange. (Reprinted with permission from *Physiology of Respiration*, by J. H. Comroe, Jr., 2nd Ed., p. 179, Year Book Medical Publishers, Inc.: Chicago, 1974.)

dependent (lower) part of the lung. In upper zones many well-ventilated alveoli are not perfused. A third example involves positive pressure ventilation, which may restrict flow through the pulmonary capillaries in the upper alveoli. Blood flow redistribution increases the dead space volume.

C. NON-UNIFORM VENTILATION

The anatomical complexity of 300 million alveoli in the healthy lungs of man precludes absolutely uniform distribution of the inspired air. Upon inspiration the descent of the two hemidiaphragms expands the lower lobes of the lungs moreso than the upper lobes. Inspiration expands the peripheral lung tissue more than the deep tissue. The uppermost ribs are less curved, and the upper thoracic cage is less mobile. Thus, the lungs will be increased in volume more at their bases than at their apices. In the standing position the sheer weight of lung tissue and blood makes the intrapleural pressure more positive at the bottom of the thorax, i.e., less sub-atmospheric.

There are pathologic causes of non-uniform ventilation as well. Regional differences in the degree of obstruction, air trapping, elasticity, and lung expansion create a situation in a large percentage of patients with chronic pulmonary disease where poorly ventilated and hyperventilated areas may co-exist side by side. Fibrosis lowers lung compliance, and less compliant lungs inflate less for a given transpulmonary pressure difference.

PERFUSION

A. PHYSIOLOGY OF THE PULMONARY CIRCULATION

It is often stated that the cardiac output at rest averages about 5 liters/min and can rise to as much as 25 liters/min during maximum exercise. Actually, this is only half the story, because just as this quantity of blood is exiting the heart via the aorta to serve the systemic needs, so also just as much blood is exiting via the pulmonary artery en route to the lungs. There are in effect 2 hearts (right and left), each with an output of about 5 liters/min. The precision in pump rate that is essential between the two is amazingly precise. Harris and Heath have calculated that if the aortic outflow gets ahead of the pulmonary inflow by only 0.1 ml per stroke, the lungs would be drained of blood within 2 hours.

Difficulties arise when one attempts to measure the pulmonary blood volume. The best reasonable estimates place it at roughly 0.5 to 1.0 liter. Although perhaps only 70 ml of blood may be in the pulmonary capillaries at any one moment, this is spread out in a very thin layer. The numerous pulmonary capillaries, with their surface convolutions, provide an enormous surface area for gas exchange. If the lungs have a blood flow of 4,900 ml/min, this means that the alveolar capillaries will be refilled 4,900/70 = 70 times each minute. Thus, blood circulation is rapid, and mixed venous blood is quickly arterialized. Postural changes alter pulmonary flow measureably, as with the systemic blood flow. Both pulmonary blood volume, as well as cardiac output, decrease by about 27% as a result of peripheral blood pooling when one moves from the supine to the standing position.

Several dynamic features of the pulmonary vascular system make it quite different from the systemic circuit. Pulmonary blood pressure is much lower than systemic, perhaps only one sixth as much. Pulmonary arterioles do not have as much vascular tone, and hence the major pressure drop is across the pulmonary capillary bed rather than across the arterioles (Figure 8-4). If the systemic capillaries have 25% of the total systemic vascular resistance, then the pulmonary capillary bed has as much as 60% of the total pulmonary vascular resistance. Also, the pulsatile nature of flow in the lungs continues into the capillaries, whereas on the systemic side it does not occur. During exercise these pulmonary capillaries open to carry the increased blood flow. This is easily managed since most capillaries are not completely filled with blood under resting conditions.

B. CONCEPT OF SHUNT

Some blood coursing through the lungs does not pass any alveoli. This blood bypasses the opportunity of becoming oxygenated. We say it is shunted. Shunt is generally defined as that portion of the left cardiac output which has not

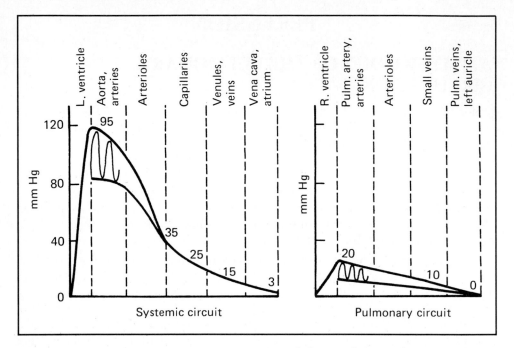

Figure 8-4. Diagrammatic representation of the cardiovascular pressures at various sites in the pulmonary and systemic circuits. There is a marked difference in the magnitude of the pressures, particularly the arterial and arteriolar, due primarily to the lowered resistance to flow and shorter length in the pulmonary circuit. (Reprinted with permission from *Physiology and Biophysics of the Circulation*, by A. C. Burton, p. 87, Year Book Medical Publishers, Inc.: Chicago, 1965.)

contacted ventilated alveoli and has not participated in gas exchange. It is quite properly termed *venous admixture.* As with dead space, shunt can be subdivided into two major components.

Anatomic shunt refers to that portion of the left cardiac output which has bypassed pulmonary capillaries, and thus has not contacted functional alveoli. There are two circulatory routes that cause this seemingly paradoxical situation in view of the usual notion of the entire cardiac output passing through the lungs. One route involves several types of vessels in the left heart which carry poorly oxygenated blood back into the left ventricle. Three types of these vessels exist. Some, called arteriosinusoidal vessels, begin as arterioles and then form irregular capillary-like sinusoids that empty into the left atrium or ventricle. Others called arterioluminal vessels connect small coronary artery branches to a heart chamber. The third group, first described in 1708 by a German physician, Adam Thebesius, allow some blood to flow from coronary veins or the ends of coronary capillaries into heart chambers. These Thebesian vessels have also been termed the venae cordis minimae. The total shunted blood volume from these routes is small. Studies by Mark Ravin indicate that perhaps no more than 0.3% of the cardiac output is comprised of Thebesian vessel blood. However, since the O_2 extraction from this shunted blood is quite high, their contribution to anatomic shunt can be sizeable.

The second route includes the drainage of lung servant tissues. The air passageways themselves, blood vessels, and lung interstitial tissue require their own special circulation using arterialized blood. The bronchial arteries serve these needs (Figure 2-9), and the venous return from the larger bronchi and pleural membranes enters the right heart via the azygos and hemiazygos veins. However, venous drainage from the smaller bronchi and bronchioles enters the pulmonary veins, which contain freshly oxygenated blood; this dilutes their O_2 content. This volume is generally less than 1% of the total left cardiac output.

Capillary shunt refers to that portion of the right cardiac output entering the pulmonary capillaries that perfuses non-ventilated alveoli. (Figure 8-5). As a result, the blood returns from these capillaries to the left heart having experienced no pulmonary gas exchange. Fluids present in the airways, pneumonia with atelectasis, destruction of lung tissue, and pulmonary edema can all contribute pathologically to capillary shunt. Oxygen therapy will not correct a shunt problem. It may increase the blood O_2 content somewhat, but unless treatment is specifically directed at alleviating the cause of the shunt, it will remain.

As a result of shunting, there is an alveolar (A) to arterial (a)O_2 gradient. That is, the P_aO_2 (alveolar PO$_2$) and $P_{LC}O_2$ (lung capillary PO$_2$), which normally equilibrate across the alveolocapillary membrane, are larger than the P_aO_2 as measured in the peripheral arterial blood. Other factors, of course, contribute to this A-a

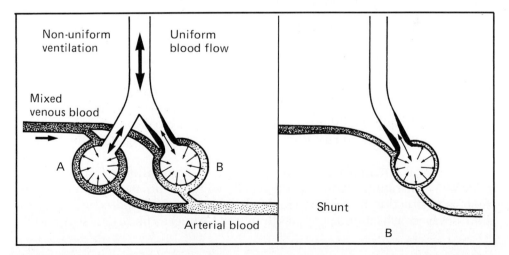

Figure 8-5. Illustration of capillary shunt, caused when a portion of the cardiac output circulates past alveoli which for some reason are inadequately ventilated. Thus, perfusion is adequate around alveoli A and B, but the poor ventilation in alveolus B decreases the functional effectiveness of these capillaries for blood gas exchange. (Reprinted with permission from *Physiology of Respiration*, by J. H. Comroe, 2nd Ed., p. 179, Year Book Medical Publishers, Inc.: Chicago, 1974.)

gradient: the alveolar PCO_2, the O_2 content of the inspired air, hemoglobin concentration, barometric pressure, and integrity of the alveolocapillary membrane. Since increased shunting increases the A-a gradient, it is useful to calculate the fraction of the cardiac output that constitutes shunted blood. The cardiac output ($\dot{Q}_t$) equals the shunted flow ($\dot{Q}_s$) plus the pulmonary capillary blood flow ($\dot{Q}_c$) which exchanges with functional alveoli. Thus, $\dot{Q}_t = \dot{Q}_c + \dot{Q}_s$. The fraction of cardiac output representing shunted bloodflow is then given by $\dot{Q}_s/\dot{Q}_t$. As an example, let us consider the case of no shunting whatever, and examine O_2 transport. The O_2 content of lung capillary blood ($C_{LC}O_2$) would equal the O_2 content of systemic arterial blood (C_aO_2). The mixed venous O_2 content ($C_{\bar{v}}O_2$) is typically 14 ml/100 ml, whereas $C_{LC}O_2$ typically is 20 ml/100 ml. The shunted O_2 content is given by $C_{LC}O_2 - C_aO_2$ and the overall arteriovenous O_2 difference is given by $C_{LC}O_2 - C_{\bar{v}}O_2$. Thus,

$$\frac{\dot{Q}_s}{\dot{Q}_t} = \frac{C_{LC}O_2 - C_aO_2}{C_{LC}O_2 - C_{\bar{v}}O_2} = \frac{20 - 20}{20 - 14} = 0$$

Even in healthy people, some shunting occurs, though no more than about 4% of the cardiac output. This is comprised almost entirely of anatomic aspects (3%).

In addition to the completely functional shunting just described, which is not improved by O_2 administration, there are two shunt-like situations that do respond to O_2 therapy. If some alveoli are poorly ventilated, or if the blood flow across ventilated alveolar surfaces is excessively rapid, a so-called *shunt effect* can result.

C. NON-UNIFORM PERFUSION

Perfusion in the lung ordinarily is non-uniform, just as ventilation is non-uniform. As a result of gravity, the column of blood in the pulmonary circulation produces a vertical hydrostatic pressure gradient in the lung blood vessels, dilating the dependent small vessels nearer the heart and increasing flow through them. Blood flow in the apex of the lung for this reason is much less than at the base. The right pulmonary artery branches off the main pulmonary trunk at a more acute angle than the left, such that momentum carries relatively more blood into the left pulmonary artery, even though the left lung is smaller than the right.

Pathological situations can also contribute to non-uniform perfusion. Any circulatory alteration producing a regional change in resistance to blood flow, such as obstruction by a blood clot (embolus), external blood vessel compression, or vasoconstriction, aggravates the normally uneven perfusion distribution.

VENTILATION/PERFUSION RATIOS AND INEQUALITIES

In order for gas exchange between alveoli and blood to occur, ventilation and perfusion must interface. The ratio of ventilation ($\dot{V}_A$) to perfusion ($\dot{Q}_c$) would be

1.0 if the matching were perfect. However, we have seen that, although all of the gas exchanging units are supplied in parallel with the same mixed venous blood (if they are capillaries) or with the identical inspired gas (if they are alveoli), the final gas composition in each alveolus prior to exhalation (and in each capillary prior to departure of blood from its proximity to alveoli) will vary widely around some mean value. This is explained by shunting and dead space.

Some general quantitation can describe this further, illustrated in *Figure 8-6*. The average resting alveolar ventilation is about 4 liters/min (the entire respiratory minute volume is about 6 liters/min), and the average pulmonary blood flow (cardiac output) is about 5 liters/min. Thus, $\dot{V}_A/\dot{Q}_c = 4/5 = 0.8$. This is the ideal situation. Absence of alveolar ventilation would result in a $\dot{V}_A/\dot{Q}_c$ ratio of 0/5, or zero, whereas absence of pulmonary capillary perfusion would produce a $\dot{V}_A/\dot{Q}_c$ ratio of 4/0, or infinity.

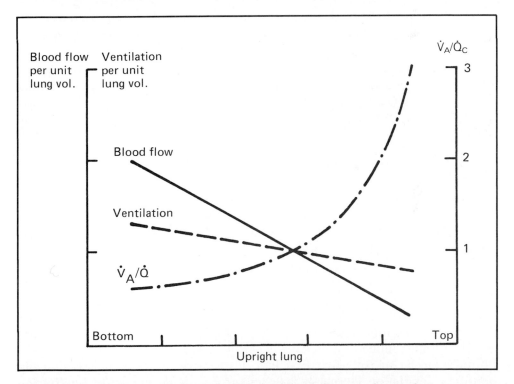

Figure 8-6. Diagram of the variation in blood flow and ventilation as one proceeds from the bottom to the top of the upright lung. Blood flow and ventilation both decrease, but not by the same amount, such that the ratio between ventilation ($\dot{V}_A$) and perfusion ($\dot{Q}_c$) is much higher near the top of the lung (3.0 or more) than near the bottom (0.8). Thus, there is overventilation relative to perfusion near the top and overperfusion relative to ventilation near the bottom. (Reprinted with permission from *Respiration in Health and Disease*, by R. M. Cherniack, L. Cherniack, and A. Naimark, p. 100, W. B. Saunders Co.: Philadelphia, 1972.)

Many ventilation/perfusion inequalities occur normally in healthy lungs. By recalling some of the examples provided earlier for nonuniform ventilation and perfusion, some perspective for this problem should already be developed. Think for a moment about the dynamics that occur as we are affected by gravity through changing of body position. If we have been recumbent, lying on our back, the posterior portion of each lung has been better perfused than ventilated (it has been in the so-called dependent position). The anterior portion has been better ventilated than perfused. If we turn over, lying on our stomach, the reverse ventilation/perfusion dominance would occur. As we stand up, the lowermost portions of the lungs will now be better perfused than ventilated.

The healthy response of the lungs to the gravitational forces imposed by such position changes is one of quick and adequate compensation. Knowledge of this can be of advantage when patients have unilateral lung disease. Clinical experience suggests that positioning the healthy lung down (toward the bed) and the diseased lung up (toward the ceiling) is often very useful for improved oxygenation. Ventilation in the diseased lung will be better, improving the changes for adequately oxygenating the blood flowing through.

Studies by J. B. West and C. T. Dollery have very nicely quantified the variation in blood flow of the healthy lung. They concluded that the mechanical pressures inside and outside the alveoli, arteries, and veins determine the flow dynamics of air and blood. Figure 8-7 illustrates how, as one moves from upper to lower regions of the lung, in the standing position, the blood flow is substantially increased. Ventilation also is altered, such that if one considers the lung as a series of thin horizontal slices, the $\dot{V}_A/\dot{Q}_c$ ratios will vary.

Such conclusions led West and his colleagues to divide the lung functionally into three zones from the standpoint of pulmonary arterial, venous, and alveolar pressures and the influences that these have on ventilation/perfusion. These zones, as well as the concepts diagrammed in Figure 8-3 and 8-5, emphasize that the lungs are by no means homogeneous in their air/blood relationships.

Zone One is the upper region of the lung, where the $\dot{V}_A/\dot{Q}_c$ ratio may range from 2.0 to more than 3.0. Here, $P_A > P_a > P_v$, because the blood vessels are collapsible and the perfusion pressure is sufficient, under routine conditions when standing, to allow pulmonary artery blood flow barely to reach the top of the lung during the maximum contraction phase of the heart (known as systole). When one lies supine, much of Zone One is perfused equally as well as Zone Two is during standing. In Zone Two, $P_a > P_A > P_v$. As alveolar pressure varies during breathing, ventilation alternately matches and does not match perfusion. During exercise, the area of the lung affected by the pressure gradients typical of Zone Two is greatly increased. In Zone Three, $P_a > P_v > P_A$ and alveolar pressure does not affect blood flow.

Since the gas-exchanging function of the lung is achieved through interaction of the ventilatory gas stream with the blood perfusing the gas-exchange regions, the $\dot{V}_A/\dot{Q}_c$ ratio has important physiologic significance. The ratio is much higher in the upper lobes (3.3) than in the lower lobes (0.55). This is a 6-fold difference.

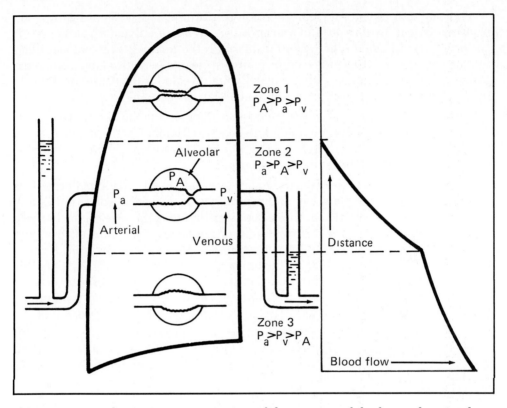

Figure 8-7.   Schematic representation of three zones of the lung, showing how differences between alveolar, arterial, and venous pressures in the three regions affect blood flow. In Zone 1 pulmonary arterial pressure can fall below alveolar pressure, and little, if any, flow will occur. In Zone 2 arterial and alveolar pressures determine flow since alveolar pressure is generally greater than venous pressure. In Zone 3 the usual arterial-venous pressure difference determines flow. (Reprinted with permission from West, J. B., Dollery, C. T., and Naimark, A., *Journal of Applied Physiology* 19:, 713, 1964.)

Because much of the ventilation and most of the blood flow goes to the middle lobes, their $\dot{V}_A/\dot{Q}_c$ ratio is much closer to the mean of 0.8.

   J. S. Haldane, in his fascinating book entitled *Respiration*, published in 1922, fully realized that an uneven distribution of ventilation or blood flow or both would produce an alveolar-arterial (A–a) pressure difference for O_2 but not necessarily for CO_2. After describing a lung that was unequally ventilated, he wrote: "The consequence of this will be that the venous blood passing through the unexpanded parts of the lung will be very imperfectly arterialized, whereas in the expanded parts the blood will be more arterialized than usual. The mixed arterial blood will thus be a mixture of over-arterialized and under-arterialized blood."

. A normal lung is a mosaic representing a continuum of gas tensions grouped in some statistical fashion around a mean value. When an alveolar gas sample is collected, it will constitute the end result of all the individual alveolocapillary interactions. Even if there may at first glance appear to be reasonably normal gas values and exchange ratios, what is usually not revealed is the degree of variance in $\dot{V}_A/\dot{Q}_c$ ratios that contributed to the alveolar gas sample.

It is the variance that is of prime importance in assessing the function of a lung. The greater this variance, the smaller must be the efficiency of the whole lung. In fact one may look at many types of pulmonary pathology as simply variable disturbances in the ventilation/perfusion ratio.

$\dot{V}_A/\dot{Q}_c$ mismatch is probably the primary cause of hypoxemia in patients. This is in contrast to hypercapnia, caused primarily by decreased alveolar ventilation. If the $\dot{V}_A/\dot{Q}_c$ ratio is low, this implies a poor ventilation of the bases of the lungs in comparison to perfusion. It can occur as a result of anesthesia, lung obstruction, obesity, pregnancy, ascites, and other problems as well. This decreased $\dot{V}_A/\dot{Q}_c$ ratio will result in hypoxemia. On the other hand, if the $\dot{V}_A/\dot{Q}_c$ ratio is high, this implies a poor perfusion of the apices compared to their ventilation. The cardiac output can be decreased as a result of shock, positive end-expiratory pressure, or left heart failure. This increased $\dot{V}_A/\dot{Q}_c$ ratio will also result in hypoxemia.

The art of good patient care requires first of all, a caring for the patient, but secondly a knowledge of the process by which health has become impaired. In the instance of ventilation and perfusion interaction, this knowledge can be challenging both to obtain and to interpret.

RELEVANT READING

Barcroft, J. *The Respiratory Function of the Blood.* Cambridge University Press, 1914.

Bohr, C. Uber die Lungenathmung. *Skandinavischen Archiv fur Physiologie* **2**:236, 1891.

Bohr, C. Uber die spezifische Tatigkeit der Lungen bei der respiratorischen Gasaufnahme. *Skandinavischen Archiv der Physiologie* **22**:221, 1909.

Bouhuys, A., and Lundin, G. Distribution of inspired gas in lungs. *Physiological Reviews* **39**:731–750, 1959.

Comroe, J. M. Jr., *Physiology of Respiration*, 2nd Ed., Chapter 13, Matching of gas and blood, pp. 168–182, Year Book Medical Publishers, Inc., Chicago, 1974.

Foster, R. E. II. The single-breath carbon monoxide transfer test 25 years on: A reappraisal. *Thorax* **38**:1–9, 1983.

Haldane, J. S., and Priestley, J. G. The regulation of the lung ventilation. *Journal of Physiology* **32**:225, 1905.

Harris, P., and Heath D. *The Human Pulmonary Circulation.* Edinburgh: Churchill Livingstone, 1962.

Johnson, R. L., Jr., Spicer, W.S., Bishop, J. M., et al. Pulmonary capillary blood volume, flow, and diffusing capacity during exercise. *Journal of Applied Physiology* **15**:893–902, 1960.

Krogh, M. The diffusion of gases through the lungs of man. *Journal of Physiology (London)* **49**:271–300, 1914–1915.

Lenfant, C. Measurement of ventilation/perfusion distribution with alveolar-arterial differences. *Journal of Applied Physiology* **18**:1090–1094, 1963.

Murray, J. F. *The Normal Lung*, Chapter 7: Gas exchange and oxygen transport, pp. 171–197. Philadelphia: W. B. Saunders Co., 1976.

Ravin, M. B., Epstein, R. M., and Malm, J. R. Contribution of thebesian veins to the physiologic shunt in anesthetized man. *Journal of Applied Physiology* **20**:1148–1152, 1965.

Rohrer, F. Der Stromungswiderstand in den menschlichen Atemwegen. *Pfluger's Archiv des gesamte Physiologie* 162:225, 1915.

Rossier, P. H., and Buhlmann, A. The respiratory dead space. *Physiological Reviews* **35**:860–876, 1955.

Wagner, P. D., and West, J. B. Effects of diffusion impairment on O_2 and CO_2 time courses in pulmonary capillaries. *Journal of Applied Physiology* **33**:62–71, 1972.

West, J. B., and Dollery, C. T. Distribution of blood flow and the pressure-flow relations of the whole lung. *Journal of Applied Physiology* **20**:175–183, 1965.

West, J. B. *Ventilation/Blood Flow and Gas Exchange*, 2nd Ed. Blackwell: Oxford, 1970.

Zuntz, N. Physiologie der Blutgase und des respiratorischen Gaswechsels. *Hermann's Handbuch der Physiologie* **4**:1, 1882.

Gas Transport in the Blood

Chapter Nine

Chapter Nine Outline

Physiology of Blood, Erythrocytes, and Hemoglobin

    A. Blood

    B. The Erythrocyte

    C. Hemoglobin

        1. The Physiologic Need for Hemoglobin

        2. Absence of Hemoglobin in Some Vertebrates

        3. Structure of the Hemoglobin Molecule

Transport of Oxygen Through the Blood

    A. Oxygen Stores in the Body and Blood

    B. Hemoglobin Binding Affinity for Oxygen

    C. Effects of Carbon Dioxide on Hemoglobin-Oxygen Interaction

    D. The Concept of P_{50}

    E. The Role of 2,3-DPG in Oxygen Dissociation

Transport of Carbon Dioxide In the Blood

    A. Modes of Transport

    B. Effects of Oxygen on Hemoglobin-CO_2 Interaction

A primary reason for the existence of the cardiovascular system is to ensure that nutrients and wastes are delivered to and removed from the living tissues via circulating blood. In this context, O_2 is a nutrient, CO_2 a waste product. Gas transport occurs not only by physical dissolution of the gases in blood, but also by their chemical combination with hemoglobin in the erythrocytes. There are four major interacting O_2 transport systems: 1) the lungs with their alveoli, 2) the blood with its hemoglobin, 3) the circulatory system with its capillaries, cardiac output, blood pressure and blood volume, and 4) the tissues with their mitochondria. It is appropriate initially in discussing gas transport functions of the blood to learn about the physiology of erythrocytes and hemoglobin as a preface to pursuing the details of how respiratory gases use these in their movement to and from the lungs and tissues. Hemoglobin fits all the most rigorous requirements that could be given to a candidate molecule for the awesome task of carrying life-ensuring quantities of O_2. It has a large capacity for O_2 in comparison to plasma, it can carry several O_2 molecules per molecule of itself, it can release O_2 upon demand, it can load and unload O_2 quickly over a PO_2 range appropriate to that found in tissues, and it can alter its binding affinity for O_2 appropriately when demands for O_2 change.

It is one of the most amazing molecules in the universe in possessing these properties. An additional function is to account for more than two-thirds of the total blood buffering of acidity in healthy humans. The study of how hemoglobin functions is one of the most fascinating topics in science.

PHYSIOLOGY OF BLOOD, ERYTHROCYTES, AND HEMOGLOBIN

A. BLOOD

From the standpoint of evolutionary time, blood in the form that we know it—a fluid serving as a transport medium—is a reasonably advanced phenomenon. If one thinks back along the phylogenetic tree to species like sponges or anemones, these survive perfectly well by allowing sea water to percolate through channels in their interior. This allows O_2 and nutrients to enter, CO_2 and wastes to leave.

The evolution of more advanced forms, with an increasing specialization of cells and an increasing body size, made necessary a more precisely regulated flow of body fluid. Hence, there arose a closed system of tubes with a pump and a precisely regulated fluid within. The blood, and the other body fluids either derived from blood or regulated by it, replace the watery sea environment that bathed the primitive creatures less sophisticated in evolutionary development. Indeed the composition of the two are rather similar, blood being slightly less osmolar than sea water.

Blood flowing through the vessels consists, under normal conditions, of a straw-colored fluid called plasma; suspended in it are two general cell types, erythrocytes and leukocytes. In addition, there are some cytoplasmic bits called platelets which have an important role in blood coagulation. The presence of these components makes its viscosity from 5 to 6 times more than that of water. The specific gravity of blood is also greater than that for water, actually rather close to that of sea water. Plasma is well buffered, in particular with bicarbonate, phosphate, and proteins, and its pH is kept at about 7.40.

The fluid component comprises about 55% of the total blood volume, and includes many groups of substances. There are dissolved respiratory gases—O_2 and CO_2. There are dozens of ions from dissociated acids, bases, and salts—Na^+, K^+, Cl^-, HCO_3^-, Ca^{++}, SO_4^-, PO_4^- just to name a few. There are all the nonprotein internal secretions, such as heparin (a naturally-occurring anti-coagulant) and steroid hormones. There are a myriad of proteins, collectively termed plasma proteins. And there are a large variety of nonprotein substances, such as glucose, triglycerides, urea, cholesterol, and bilirubin. All these are in a water medium, water comprising the vast majority of the total plasma volume. Some of these substances may be water-insoluble, such as cholesterol and the steroid hormones, but they are solubilized by binding to proteins.

The plasma proteins are many in number and equally diverse in function. CO_2 can be transported on any of them possessing the amino acid valine at the end of their molecular structures. Albumin comprises the largest fraction of the plasma proteins and is responsible for most of the osmotic balance occurring between blood and other fluids. Fibrinogen is involved in blood clotting, and it is this protein that creates the primary difference between plasma and serum. Serum is the straw-colored fluid resulting when blood is allowed to clot, and the clot removed. Plasma is the fluid portion of non-clotted blood, and thus still contains fibrinogen.

A large group of proteins includes the globulins, which have an integral role in immune reactions. Other plasma proteins are responsible for binding lipids (lipoproteins) and nonsoluble hormones (sex-steroid binding globulin is one example). Still others are enzymes.

The solid component of blood contains all of the cells and cell fragments. It makes up the other 45% of the total volume; this value is termed the hematocrit. It is normally a little lower (42) in females than in males (45). Prior to puberty, the erythrocyte count in males is the same as in females; it is increased after puberty in males as a result of rising levels of anabolic hormones that eventually stimulate the bone marrow to release more erythrocytes into the bloodstream.

Although the term hematocrit strictly refers to the percent of erythrocytes by volume, since the total leukocyte and platelet count are so small by comparison, they are often included with the erythrocytes in determination of hematocrit. These cells form a "buffy coat" at the erythrocyte-plasma interface when the blood is centrifuged. Typically in one cubic millimeter (mm^3) of blood there are 5,400,000 erythrocytes (in men, 4,800,000 in women), 7,000 leukocytes, and 250,000 platelets. Since 1 ml = 1 cc = 1,000 mm^3, each of these values must be multiplied by 1,000 to represent the number of cells or platelets per ml of blood.

With a composition so varied, one would expect that the functions of blood would be equally diverse. Indeed they are, and although we are interested here only in one or two of them, several should be listed to provide perspective as to the importance of this fluid:

1. to supply food in a dissolved state from the alimentary canal to the other tissues;
2. to remove waste products of metabolism;
3. to stabilize body temperature and water levels;
4. to allow gaseous exchange with the environment—O_2 from the environment to the interior, and CO_2 in the reverse direction; and
5. to form a barrier to invasion by injurious processes, using at least three mechanisms:
   a. antigen-antibody reactions, principally involving the plasma proteins and leukocytes;
   b. inflammatory and allergic reactions, utilizing leukocytes; and
   c. clotting reactions, involving platelets, erythrocytes, and plasma proteins.

B. THE ERYTHROCYTE

This cell functions primarily as a transport vehicle for hemoglobin. If hemoglobin were carried in the plasma, the blood would be much more viscous, requiring additional work for its circulation. By concentrating hemoglobin into small packages (erythrocytes), the overall blood viscosity is minimized. Mammalian erythrocytes have no nuclei, unlike those of amphibians, fish, reptiles, and birds, thus cannot divide. Nevertheless, they are metabolically active, with all the enzymes present to permit glycolysis.

There is no direct relationship between body size and erythrocyte size: the cells of moles, man, and elephants are similar in size to all other mammals. The typical mammalian erythrocyte shape is that of a biconcave disc (Figure 9-1), measuring about 7 μm × 2 μm (the camel is unique with oval discs). It contains about 66% water and 33% hemoglobin by volume. The cell shape appears optimal for the combined requirements of: 1) maximal surface area for diffusion of gases; 2) minimal surface tension changes when the cell changes volume; and 3) great capacity to be deformed without losing structural integrity.

As erythrocytes move from arterial to venous blood, via capillaries that often are half their diameter, the actions of hemoglobin as a buffer bring about a gradual increase in intracellular osmolarity. To balance this change, the cells enlarge somewhat, and bulge as water moves in. The volume increase will be from 2% to 5%. After the cells transit through the lungs, the arterial shape returns as water exits and pH balance is restored. Excessive expansion of the cell volume can result in hemolysis via cell rupture.

Such cell volume changes alter the rheological properties of blood, which in turn changes blood viscosity. This is partially overcome by the unique properties

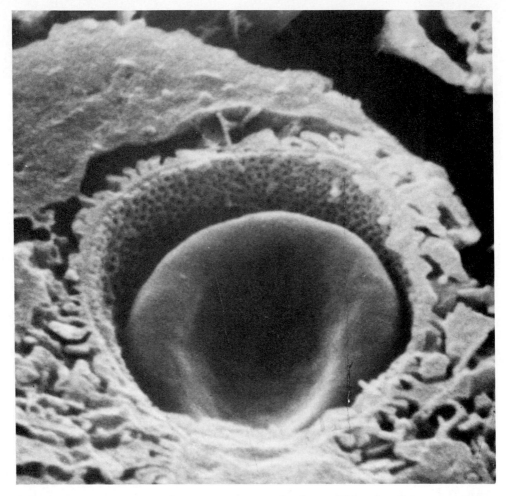

Figure 9-1. Scanning electron micrograph of a red blood cell in a capillary. Notice that the diameters of both are rather similar. In many instances the red blood cell can course through even smaller capillaries. This is made possible because the cells are deformable, thanks in large measure to their biconcave disc shape.

of hemoglobin molecules within erythrocytes. Their mechanical properties alternate between those of a sol and a gel, depending upon whether external forces influencing flow are increased or decreased. Blood with a hematocrit of 100% still retains fluid properties, which is of great benefit with flow under extreme conditions such as hemoconcentration. During prolonged exercise in hot weather, when venous volume is reduced through water loss from perspiration, energy-efficient flow in this more viscous blood is still ensured.

Where are erythrocytes produced? This varies with the age of the individual. As seen in *Figure 9-2*, during the first few weeks of embryonic life, the yolk sac is chiefly responsible. As pregnancy ensues, this function is gradually shifted to the liver and later on to the spleen. At about the fifth to sixth month of pregnancy, the bone marrow begins to become highly specialized for this task. After delivery, erythrocyte production rapidly becomes the primary function of bone marrow. Through adolescence most bones have erythrocyte-producing marrow in them. After adulthood, the vertebrae, sternum, ribs, pelvis and upper portions of each humerus and femur remain the primary sources.

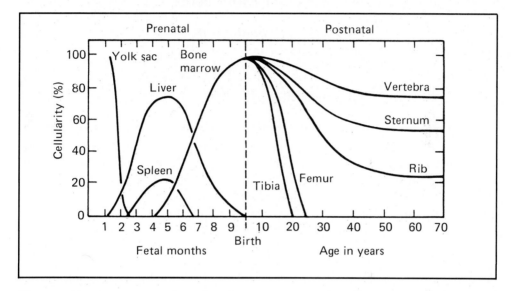

Figure 9-2. Diagram to show the changing sites utilized by the body for production of red blood cells during fetal life, and the relative restriction of such erythropoietic activity, following birth, to marrow cavities within certain bones. (Reprinted with permission from Erslev, A.J., and Weiss, L. "Structure and Function of the Marrow." Chapter 12 in *Hematology*, (W.J. Williams, E. Beutler, A.J. Erslev, and M.A. Lichtman, eds.), 3rd Ed., p. 75, McGraw-Hill Book Co.: New York, 1983).

How are erythrocytes produced? These cells are the end result of a long line of cell types, differentiating from primitive stem cells in the marrow *(Figure 9-3)*. The mechanism which triggers a primitive stem cell to begin its maturation is unknown at present. It is known that hypoxia—lowered tissue O_2 supply—from whatever cause—be it anemia, a sojourn to altitudes above about 5,000 feet (1,868 meters), or blood loss through a wound or hemorrhaging—can accelerate the process. The initial stages in the complex cell differentiation process divide, but the later stages do not. It appears that the gradually increasing synthesis of hemoglobin in these cell types controls this division.

The kidney is of primary regard in responding to this hypoxia, and responds by increasing circulating blood levels of a hormone called renal erythropoietic erythropoietin. This substance actively influences the bone marrow to increase

Committed stem cell
↓
Large Basophilic Normoblast (E_1)
↓
Small Basophilic Normoblast (E_2)
↓
Polychromatophilic Normoblast (E_4)
↓
Late Dividing Normoblast (E_5)
↓
Reticulocyte (E_6)
↓
Erythrocyte (E_7)

Figure 9-3.   Stages in the differentiation of committed primitive bone marrow stem cell populations into mature red blood cells. No further cell division occurs beyond E_5, presumably because accumulation of sizable quantities of hemoglobin suppresses such activity. Reticulocytes and erythrocytes have no nuclei. Reticulocytes are primarily marrow-dwellers, but can be found in the blood when the proliferation process is increased in intensity.

its rate of release of mature erythrocytes into the bloodstream. (Testosterone will increase the quantities of erythropoietin as part of its anabolic protein building activities.) The effect of erythropoietin on the bone marrow is usually limited by available iron. An increase in erythrocyte production can reach about twice the basal value—from a daily rate of 1% of the circulating erythrocyte mass to about 2%.

Once produced and circulating, erythrocytes do not have an easy time in maintaining their existence. They are forced through capillaries which can be as small as 4 μm in diameter—less than half of their own cellular diameter! This feat is achieved through their enormous deformability, permissible as a result of the great surface area-to-volume ratio caused by their biconcave shape. Realizing that viscosity of blood, determined in large measure by erythrocyte cell shape, is an important determinant in blood flow, it is easy to see how gas transport through highly active tissues is also closely related to the metabolic state of these cells.

After a lifespan of about 120 days, erythrocytes are unable to endure the rigors of another circuit through the bloodstream, and they disintegrate. Some approximate calculations provide an interesting perspective on the kinetics of this process. Using a mean erythrocyte count of $5 \times 10^6/mm^3$, and an average circulating blood volume of 70 ml/kg body weight, this represents 350×10^9 erythrocytes/kg body weight. Assuming a mean erythrocyte lifespan of 120 days, there must be an average of $(350 \times 10^9)/120 = 2.9 \times 10^9$ erythrocytes/kg produced daily. This is a production of 3,350 erythrocytes per kg/sec. If equilibrium is to be maintained, then a similar number must be destroyed.

Erythrocyte destruction results in the liberation of hemoglobin into the surrounding plasma. This occurs primarily in the spleen. The hemoglobin is converted into its two chief constituents, heme and globin. The heme portion loses its iron atoms and is converted first into the green pigment called biliverdin and later into the orange pigment bilirubin (Figure 9-4). The iron is quite valuable and will be retained in the liver, spleen, and elsewhere for re-use in hemoglobin synthesis. Bilirubin is a true waste product. The liver excretes bilirubin through the large intestine via the gall bladder. Excreted bilirubin thus contributes to fecal coloration. Hepatic malfunction can cause a pigmentation of the skin and other tissues as a result of bilirubin buildup in the blood. This condition is termed icterus or jaundice.

C. HEMOGLOBIN

1. The Physiologic Need for Hemoglobin

Metabolizing tissues require quantities of O_2 which are far in excess of those solely dissolved in the bloodstream. Thus, a reservoir of bound, or stored, O_2 is mandatory. Hemoglobin serves these needs admirably. Although hemoglobin has additional important roles in transport of CO_2 and hydrogen ions, which makes it an important buffer against acidosis, its role as an O_2 reservoir is of primary importance.

A better appreciation for this role is provided by examining in greater detail the O_2 needs of the body. Some simple calculations can be made using standardized conditions. These represent ideal situations. For example, when gas partial pressures are determined in blood, standard barometric pressure of 760 mmHg (13.3 kPa) is used to relate the quantity dissolved in terms of a dry gas gradient.

At rest, a 70 kg individual will extract between 5 and 6 ml of O_2 per 100 ml of blood (0.23 to 0.28 mM/L). This is determined indirectly by use of the principle identified in the nineteenth century by the German physician Adolph Fick. He realized that the blood flow to an organ could be expressed as the ratio of that organ's uptake of a given substance to the organ's removal of the substance. If the entire body is the "organ" under consideration, with O_2 the substance used, then the blood flow becomes the left ventricular cardiac output (CO), which averages 5,000 ml/min, the tissue O_2 utilization becomes the basal volume of O_2 consumption ($\dot{V}O_2$), which averages about 250 ml/min, (11.3 mM/min), and the O_2 removed is the difference between the mixed venous O_2 and the arterial O_2. This a–v O_2 difference then can be calculated as $\dot{V}O_2/CO = 250/5,000 = 0.05$ ml O_2/ml blood, or 5 ml O_2/100 ml blood (11.3/5,000 = 0.0023 mM/ml).

Henry's law (Chapter Eight) indicates that the dissolution of O_2 in the blood is a fairly linear relationship. Thus, at the typically observed P_aO_2 of 100 mmHg (13.3 kPa), the dissolved blood O_2 content is 0.3 ml/100 ml (0.14 mM/L). If the PO_2 is reduced by a factor of 10 (10 mmHg, 1.3 kPa), then the blood could contain 0.03

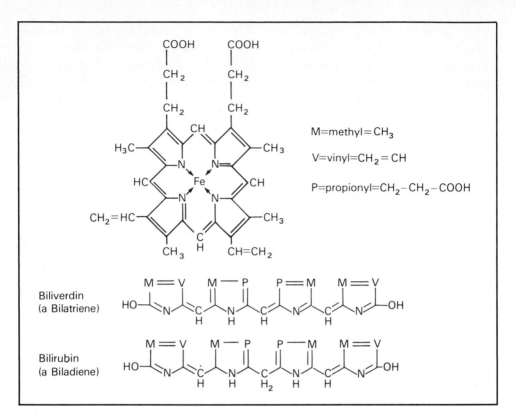

Figure 9-4. Chemical formulas for heme, and two of its metabolic breakdown products, biliverdin and bilirubin. Chemically, the heme molecule is a tetrapyrrole ring structure, which can bind not only to iron but also to the protein globin. A hemoglobin molecule is comprised of four such heme/iron/globin units. When erythrocytes break down, and their hemoglobin is released into the plasma, it is systematically degraded. Breaking of the heme ring at the point indicated releases iron (which is conserved by the body) and leaves the long-chain compound biliverdin. This is subsequently further hydrogenated into bilirubin. Both are waste products and excreted through the large intestine.

ml O_2/100 ml (0.014 mM/L). Raising the PO_2 to 1000 mmHg (133 kPa) increases the dissolved O_2 to 3 ml/100 ml (1.4 mM/L). Thus, for the blood to carry 6 ml O_2/100 ml blood (0.27 mM/L), which would provide the essential 5 ml/100 ml (0.23 mM/L) as well as a small reserve, a P_aO_2 of 2,000 mmHg (266 kPa) would be required. It is quite impossible to achieve this on Earth except in man-made hyperbaric chambers.

The only other possible means for ensuring adequate O_2 to the tissues, apart from raising the PO_2, would be to increase the volume of tissue blood flow. A few additional calculations reveal why such an increase would also be impossible. A 70 kg person consuming 3.5 ml O_2/kg body weight/min (0.158 mM O_2) will require $70 \times 3.5 = 245$ ml O_2/kg/min ($70 \times 0.158 = 11.1$ mM O_2). Perfusing blood containing 0.3 ml O_2/100 ml (0.14 mM/L) would need to flow at 245/3.0 = 81.7 L/min to provide this requirement (11.1/0.14 = 79.3 L/min). This is approximately 80/5 = 16 times more than the resting left ventricular cardiac output. Clearly then, the hemoglobin as a reservoir for O_2 transport is extremely effective.

2. Absence of Hemoglobin in some Vertebrates

It might seem almost inconceivable that any species of vertebrate could exist without hemoglobin or a related O_2-binding molecule. Any vertebrate form that could exist without hemoglobin must be restricted to a very unique geographical environment (where O_2 concentration is high) and have unique adaptations for survival.

About two dozen species of fish live in the frigid (2°C) waters of the Antarctic Ocean. They are typified by the Antarctic icefish *(Chaenocephalus aceratus)*. Their body is almost devoid of scales, allowing O_2 to penetrate rather easily through the skin as well as through the gills. There is a well-developed cutaneous circulation, and their slender body, as long as two feet, has a high ratio of surface area to mass. The fish are poikilothermic (cold-blooded) and live in frigid water. Their surrounding sea water as well as their circulating blood contains about 50% more O_2 than water or hemoglobin-free blood at 20°C. The basal metabolic rate of these fish is about one-sixth that of fish of comparable size living at 20°C. They do have bone marrow, which produces leukocytes, and according to some reports, a small number of erythrocytes (fewer than leukocytes). But these contribute negligibly to the total O_2 carrying ability of the blood.

Although all these adaptations to survival without hemoglobin may be effective, it is interesting to speculate whether the absence of hemoglobin could in fact be of selective advantage. David Pierson has advanced the notion that "in the twilight of an Antarctic kelp forest it is harder to see the ice fish than a normally-pigmented fish. The ice fish may thus be more successful at surprising prey and eluding predators without hemoglobin." Such speculation is quite intriguing, and forms one of the fascinations of comparative respiratory physiology.

3. Structure of the Hemoglobin Molecule

The globin portion of hemoglobin is comprised of four polypeptide chains, two α and two β. About 96% of the total weight of hemoglobin is accounted for by globin. Various forms of hemoglobin are characterized by the specific chemistry of the globin chains. Thus, hemoglobin A_1, forming 90% of that seen in adults, has one pair of α chains (each containing 141 amino acids), and one pair of β chains (146 amino acids). Hemoglobin A_2 has one pair of δ chains substituted for two β chains; it constitutes another 2½% of adult hemoglobin (HbA). Fetal hemoglobin (HbF), which can represent as much as 85% of the total in a newborn infant, has one pair of γ chains replacing two β chains of HbA. Both δ and γ chains have 146 amino acids; the former is variant from β chain composition by only 8 amino acids, the latter is markedly altered. Fourteen percent of the dietary protein intake each day is incorporated into the synthesis of globin, which amounts to about 8 grams.

There are many hemoglobin-like molecules found in species throughout the animal kingdom, so it is likely that these all evolved along parallel lines. It was the substitution of iron for magnesium in the basic structure of chlorophyll that allowed hemoglobin to form, thus paving the way for the organic evolution of animals. The redox (oxidation/reduction) reactions made possible by the use of iron in the cytochrome enzymes could never have been possible if magnesium had been retained. However, in blood, when O_2 reacts with iron in hemoglobin, there are no such redox reactions. Rather, the molecule simply becomes oxygenated or de-oxygenated, and iron remains in the ferrous ($+2$) state.

The structure of hemoglobin gives many clues as to how it acts in carrying respiratory gases. It is a roughly spherical molecule with dimensions of $64 \times 55 \times 50$ Ångstroms. One 12-Ångstrom-diameter heme group is positioned in a shallow crevice of each of the four globin protein chains. Heme is the central building block for hemoglobin, and derived from the porphyrin ring (Figure 9-4), present in almost all cells. It is related closely to the structure of the cytochromes which also are found in nearly all aerobic tissue, a major difference being in the oxidation state of iron ($+2$ in heme, $+3$ in cytochromes). It is the iron atom that links the tetrapyrrole ring to the globin portion of the molecule, attaching to a specific histidine residue. With hemoglobin A_1 this is amino acid position 87 of the α chain and position 92 of the β chain.

Each globin polypeptide chain is under the control of a separate gene in the DNA of primitive erythrocytes. Mutations in DNA can result in mutant polypeptide sequences; about 100 of these have been isolated. Most are not physiologically debilitating because they do not adversely affect the shape of the hemoglobin molecule. One exception is noteworthy. In sickle cell anemia, the sixth amino acid on the β chains, normally glutamic acid, is replaced by valine. Thus, out of 574 amino acids, only two are altered from the normal adult hemoglobin pattern. Valine is hydrophobic, while glutamic acid is hydrophilic. Sickle cell hemoglobin (HbS) thus has physical properties that are affected by this influence of valine, which are quite different from normal adult hemoglobin. Upon de-oxygenation it gels into liquid crystals which are spindle shaped and rigid. These crystals deform the erythrocyte into a characteristic sickle appearance, increasing its fragility and shortening its life span. The increased rate of hemolysis causes anemia.

Those individuals who have sickle cell trait, that is, a mixture of HbS and HbA, do not exhibit the sickling hemolysis except at higher altitude, and during vigorous exercise. The incidence of this trait among American blacks is about 8% to 10%. The trait by itself confers neither a selective advantage nor disadvantage during reproductive years, so its frequency probably will not change. Those with sickle cell disease (HbS alone) experience sickling at in vivo O_2 partial pressures.

The high incidence of sickle cell trait in nations stretching from India to West Africa results from an increased resistance to infection with the unicellular protozoan *Plasmodium falciparum*, which causes malaria. Part of the life cycle of this parasite occurs in the erythrocytes. When mosquitoes of the genus *Anopheles*, which carry the protozoan, inject this organism into the human bloodstream, it eventually resides in the liver, where it subsequently divides into the next form of its life cycle. This form, called the merozooite, re-enters the bloodstream, invades erythrocytes and uses the amino acids of hemoglobin as well as ATP, glucose, and other available substances, to grow and multiply. Eventually, a few dozen merozooites are formed by nuclear division, and these leave the erythrocyte as the life cycle continues. It is the release of these merozooites that brings about the dreaded malarial fever.

The much-reduced life span of sickle cells, with their subsequent removal and destruction of the merozooites contained within, keeps the disease within manageable limits by preventing merozooite multiplication into numbers sufficient to induce fever. Thus, the advantage of having a heterozygotic population (HbS and HbA) with malaria and sickle cell trait balances the disadvantage of a homozygotic population (HbS) with sickle cell anemia.

The molecular weight of hemoglobin A_1 is 64,458 daltons. Knowing this, one can calculate the O_2 carrying capacity of hemoglobin. One gram mole carries 4 gram moles of O_2, since there are 4 binding sites, one on each heme moiety. One gram mole of O_2 represents 22,400 ml of O_2, and this would be transported by $64,458/4 = 16,115$ gm of hemoglobin. The O_2 carried by each gram of hemoglobin is then $22,400/16,115 = 1.39$ ml. This is a theoretical value, and in reality the observed O_2 carrying capacity is closer to 1.31 ml/gm. Quite often, in clinical practice the quantity of 1.34 ml/gm is used.

Myoglobin is a related O_2 carrying pigment, with only one heme moiety and a globin chain of 153 amino acids. Its molecular weight is about 17,000, and it binds only one O_2 molecule. Its affinity for O_2 is much higher than that of hemoglobin, the significance of which will become clear shortly.

TRANSPORT OF OXYGEN THROUGH THE BLOOD

A. OXYGEN STORES IN THE BODY AND BLOOD

We have seen that O_2 is found in four forms in the body: 1) as a gas in the lungs; 2) as dissolved O_2 in tissue fluids; 3) as oxyhemoglobin in blood; and 4) as oxymyoglobin in muscle. In contrast to CO_2, the stores of O_2 are really quite small and must continually be replenished for life to continue. As we shall see, most of the O_2 is chemically bound, either to hemoglobin or myoglobin, both of which have a high binding affinity for O_2. This affinity keeps most of the O_2 from being liberated into the tissues—except when badly needed—and then it moves with ease because of special mechanisms which we shall discuss.

Stopping the circulation to tissues initiates more rapid changes than those seen with stopping of breathing. Some tissues, such as skeletal and cardiac muscle, have myoglobin, and thus are protected. Although the O_2 bound to oxymyoglobin is present in the relatively low concentration of about 1 ml O_2/100 ml muscle tissue, this reservoir extends that tissue's survival time to about 3 minutes before its O_2 supply is critically low. Brain tissue, however, is quite vulnerable. This tissue requires about 5 ml O_2/min/100 gm, and its capillary blood volume is about 6 ml/100 gm. The critical PO_2 for brain aerobic metabolism can be reached in under 4 seconds.

Not only do O_2 requirements vary widely among individual tissues in any given species, but also there is an enormous variation among species. A crayfish requires 0.78 ml O_2/kg/min, a resting butterfly 10 ml/kg/min, and a flying butterfly 1,670 ml/kg/min. Resting humans by comparison require 2.5 ml/kg/min, but their myocardium requires 16 ml/kg/min. Elite distance runners can consume as much as 80 ml/kg/min, but for a period lasting no longer than a few minutes.

Several calculations can be made which characterize O_2 transport in the human bloodstream, using baseline information. Let us assume that one gm of hemoglobin combines chemically with 1.31 ml of O_2, and that every 100 ml of blood in a healthy man typically contain 15 gm of hemoglobin (13 gm in women). The arterial blood PO_2 of a healthy subject at rest is about 100 mmHg (13.3 kPa). At this P_aO_2, the hemoglobin molecules are about 97% saturated with O_2.

From these facts, and O_2 solubility information discussed earlier (Chapter Eight), the total dissolved O_2 in 100 ml of arterial blood [P_aO_2 = 100 mmHg (13.3 kPa)] is calculated as 0.003 × 100 = 0.30 ml/100 ml. Bound O_2 is calculated as hemoglobin concentration × binding affinity × % hemoglobin saturation = 15 × 1.31 × 0.97 = 19.06 ml/100 ml for men and 13 × 1.31 × 0.97 = 16.52 ml/100 ml for women.

The total O_2 content of the arterial blood is the sum of the dissolved and bound O_2. In the examples used above, this would be 0.30 + 19.06 = 19.36 ml/100 ml for men and 0.30 + 16.52 = 16.82 ml/100 ml for women. Thus, the bound O_2 constitutes 98.5% of the total O_2 carried in the blood of a healthy male, and 98.2% of that in a healthy female. If we approximate the systemic arterial O_2 delivery in man as 20 ml O_2/100 ml blood, and assume the output of the left heart as 5,000 ml/min, then it can be seen that systemic arterial O_2 transport is on the order of 1,000 ml/min.

After blood has circulated systemically, and has returned to the right ventricle, ready for transport to the lungs and oxygenation, it will have given up a sizeable portion of its available O_2 for tissue metabolism. The PO_2 of this mixed venous blood is typically 40 mmHg (5.3 kPa), and the hemoglobin molecules are still about 75% saturated. The total dissolved O_2 in 100 ml of venous blood can be calculated as 40 × 0.003 = 0.12 ml/100 ml. The total bound O_2 in 100 ml of venous blood, assuming the same hemoglobin concentrations as used in the examples above, would be 15 × 1.31 × 0.75 = 14.74 ml/100 ml for men and 13 × 1.31 × 0.75 = 12.77 ml/100 ml for women. In venous blood, the bound O_2 constitutes (14.74/14.86) × 100 = 99.2% of the total transported O_2 in men (and an almost identical 99.1% of the total in women.)

From a pulmonary point of view it is very important to assess the ability of the lungs to raise alveolar and pulmonary capillary PO_2 to a value where mixed venous blood can be adequately oxygenated. Because hemoglobin predominates in terms of quantity of O_2 transported, the percent saturation of hemoglobin with O_2 is the key parameter involved in assessment of lung oxygenating ability. A measure of O_2 content in the blood can be misleading.

As an example, consider a male patient who is anemic, with 9 gm of hemoglobin per ml blood, who has no pulmonary problems, and has a normal hemoglobin saturation of 97%. This patient's total O_2 content, as determined by the sum of dissolved and bound O_2, would be $0.30 + (8 \times 1.31 \times 0.97) = 0.30 + 10.17 = 10.47$ ml/100 ml blood. This is a 45% reduction in O_2 content from that measured in a healthy male, with healthy lungs. If this anemic patient's lungs were also diseased, his O_2 content would be further reduced, because of a smaller quantity of O_2 bound to hemoglobin.

B. HEMOGLOBIN BINDING AFFINITY FOR OXYGEN

In contrast to the dissolved O_2, which relates linearly to the PO_2 to which the blood is exposed, the O_2 associated with hemoglobin is not linearly related. *Figure 9-5* illustrates what happens to the percent saturation of hemoglobin when the PO_2 to which it is exposed is increased from 0 to 100 mmHg (0 to 13.3 kPa). The curve is S-shaped with a steep slope between 10 and 50 mmHg PO_2 (1.3 to 6.7 kPa), and a flat portion in the range of 70 to 100 mmHg (9.3 to 13.3 kPa). Memorization of four sets of values allows a general reconstruction of the curve: 25% and 15 mmHg (2 kPa), 50% and 25 mmHg (3.3 kPa), 75% and 40 mmHg (5.3 kPa), and 97% and 100 mmHg (13.3 kPa).

It should be clear that the lung oxygenating system for hemoglobin is efficient. As mentioned in Chapter Eight (see *Figure 8-1*), blood is typically exposed to alveolar gas for just under one second. In that short time, hemoglobin is brought to 97% saturation with O_2. Thus, there is little need for the blood to have longer exposure to alveolar gas. In fact, 0.25 second is normally all that is required. At a PO_2 of 100 mmHg (13.3 kPa), equilibration between any functional alveolus and its functional capillary will occur in 100 msec.

The mechanism by which O_2 binds to hemoglobin is quite interesting. The polypeptide globin chains are folded in such a way that the heme moieties fit in a kind of pocket. O_2 can readily bind without altering the volume of the molecule. Oxygenation of the first heme group of an unoxygenated hemoglobin molecule increases the binding affinity of the other heme groups. Initially, this was termed a heme-heme interaction, but modern terminology refers to it as a homotropic interaction. It is this kind of interaction that explains the sigmoid shape of the oxyhemoglobin dissociation curve. That portion of the curve at very low PO_2 values represents the initial loading of hemoglobin with O_2. The steepest portion represents the binding of two more O_2 molecules, and the flat portion at still higher PO_2 values represents loading of the final O_2 molecule.

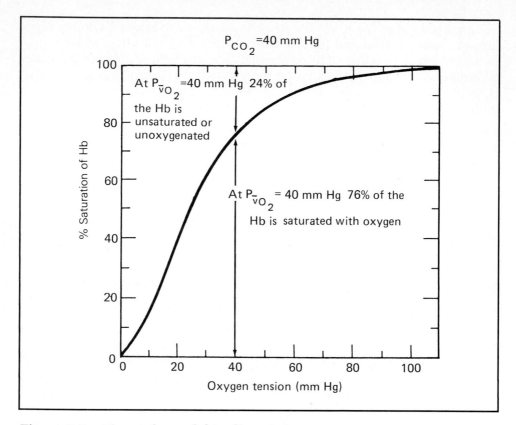

Figure 9-5. The oxyhemoglobin dissociation curve.

This same principle occurs with unloading of O_2 from hemoglobin as the PO_2 to which it is exposed falls from 100 mmHg (13.3 kPa). The hemoglobin molecule changes shape slightly, the 2 β subunits moving apart by about 6.5 Ångstroms, and the 2 α heme moieties coming together by about 1 Ångstrom. The shape changes are made possible by the alternate forming and breaking of salt bridges among the various parts of the hemoglobin molecule. It is almost as if the hemoglobin molecule itself were breathing, with oxygenation and deoxygenation alternately causing a relaxed (R) configuration when O_2 binds, and a tense (T) configuration when O_2 leaves. Such shifts in configuration occur as many as 10^8 times in the life of an erythrocyte.

There are at least 100 different mutations known which represent changes in hemoglobin structure. It seems logical that any mutations which would alter the points of contact between globin chains or between heme and globin chains would affect the R/T state stability, thus altering O_2 dissociation. It is a compelling example of how an organism's ability to survive in its environment is determined by genetic molecular biology.

The steep slope of the oxyhemoglobin dissociation curve provides for a sizable increase in the rate of O_2 release from hemoglobin should the blood PO_2 fall much below 40 mmHg (5.3 kPa). This situation is desirable. In disease states accompanied by fever, or with increased metabolism from other causes, O_2 demands will be greater than normal. The sigmoid relationship of O_2 binding to hemoglobin permits these demands to be met more easily than if the relationship were linear. An anemic patient's curve will have exactly the same shape as that of a person with normal blood composition.

Because the shape of the oxyhemoglobin dissociation curve is asymptotic from 80 to 100 mmHg (10.6 to 13.3 kPa), mammals can live at a wide range of altitudes [from sea level to 10,000 ft. (3,050 m)] with relative ease. The O_2 reservoir is large, and on one pass through the bloodstream, venous blood still has its hemoglobin well oxygenated [75% when $P_{\bar{v}}O_2$ = 40 mmHg (5.3 kPa)].

However, an understanding of the curve's shape also makes it clear that, since hemoglobin is almost saturated with O_2 during room air breathing, healthy individuals should not be able to raise their blood O_2 very much by breathing pure O_2. Assuming that the P_AO_2 could rise to 650 mmHg (86.5 kPa), and the saturation of hemoglobin with O_2 could increase to 99%, this would provide an arterial blood O_2 content of $(0.003 \times 650) + (15 \times 1.31 \times 0.99) = 1.95 + 19.45 = 21.40$ ml/100 ml. This is a mere $(21.40 - 19.36)/19.36 \times 100 = 10.5\%$ increase in blood O_2 content despite a nearly fivefold increase in O_2 content of the inspired air.

The dissociation curve for myoglobin is a hyperbola (Figure 9-6). This is explained by its single heme group, which prevents heme-heme interaction effects. It is fully saturated at a PO_2 of only 27 mmHg (3.6 kPa), and it is able to release large quantities of its bound O_2 to active muscle tissue at a PO_2 of 4 to 5 mmHg (0.5 to 0.7 kPa). Thus, muscle tissue is admirably suited to meet the needs of exercise by the interaction of hemoglobin and myoglobin, the former unloading its O_2 for entry into the cells, the latter loading the O_2 from the blood for release to muscle cell mitochondria. It is useful to think of O_2 as cascading from lungs to blood to tissues and finally to mitochondria, moving down its concentration gradient.

C. EFFECTS OF CARBON DIOXIDE ON HEMOGLOBIN-OXYGEN INTERACTION

The precise nature of the relationship between hemoglobin and O_2 was discovered by Denmark's leading physiologist at the turn of the century, Christian Bohr, and two of his students, August Krogh and Karl Hasselbalch. In their paper of 1904, they described not only the sigmoid curve, but also an unexpected strong influence of CO_2 on this binding of O_2 to hemoglobin. If the PCO_2 was increased, the entire curve was displaced to the right (Figure 9-7), to the left with a lower PCO_2. This was the first example of a heterotropic interaction, that is, the presence of one molecule (CO_2) affecting the binding of another (O_2) to a third molecule i.e., hemoglobin. An increased PCO_2 shifts the curve to the right. This increased PCO_2 can be caused by fever or exercise (both of which increase body

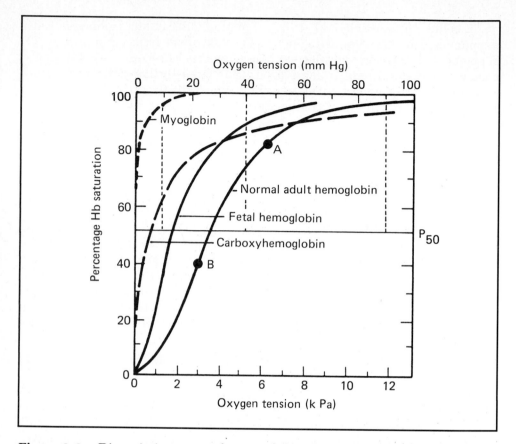

Figure 9-6. Dissociation curves for myoglobin, fetal hemoglobin, adult normal hemoglobin, and adult carboxyhemoglobin. Point A represents the PO_2 of arterial blood at which some form of beneficial oxygenation treatment must be administered unless hypoxic conditions become deleterious for general tissue function. Point B in arterial blood represents the threshold for hypoxia-induced loss of consciousness. (Redrawn with permission from *Applied Respiratory Physiology*, by J.F. Nunn, 2nd Ed., p. 403, Butterworths: London, 1977.)

metabolism. Along with CO_2 itself, the existence of H^+ ions formed from the dissociation of H_2CO_3 after the hydration of CO_2 also affects oxygen-hemoglobin affinity.

Bohr and his students realized the importance of this relationship quickly. In the tissues, the CO_2 entering capillary blood would assist hemoglobin with its unloading of O_2. Then, in the lungs, the rapid removal of CO_2 would facilitate its re-oxygenation. Thus, the essence of good tissue oxygenation is to have O_2 deliverable under an adequate partial pressure difference between blood and tissue.

The so-called Bohr shift of the oxyhemoglobin dissociation curve has important chemical significance. In man, the natural affinity of hemoglobin for O_2 is so

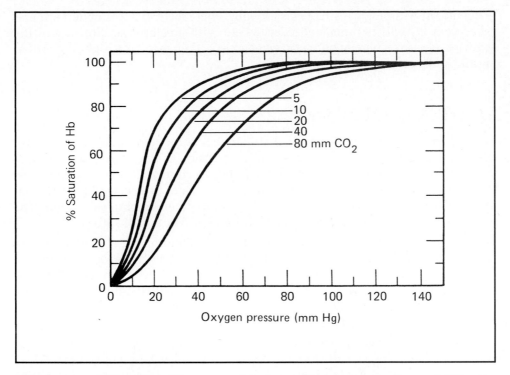

Figure 9-7. When blood is exposed to increasing concentrations of CO_2, the oxyhemoglobin dissociation curve is shifted to the right as a result of the heterotropic interaction between the two molecules (O_2 and CO_2) for hemoglobin. This relationship was demonstrated by Christian Bohr and co-workers early in the 20th century.

great that it blocks almost any release at normally-encountered PO_2 levels. This must be modified by environmental factors, of which the two most important are CO_2 and H^+ ions. Both reduce the affinity of hemoglobin for O_2 by binding as chemical ligands, CO_2 to valine moieties on the globin chains (thus forming carbamino groups), hydrogen strengthening salt bridges on the same globin chains. These ligands thus alter the shape of the hemoglobin molecule, which in turn changes the O_2 affinity. Crystals of completely deoxygenated hemoglobin are very different in appearance from those that are oxygenated. This was vividly described in 1938 by Felix Haurowitz in Prague, who exposed crystals of horse hemoglobin to O_2 while observing them microscopically. The formation of oxyhemoglobin crystals from deoxyhemoglobin was beautiful and unforgettable.

A decrease in the capillary pH from 7.4 to 7.3 at a capillary PO_2 of 40 mmHg (5.3 kPa) will decrease the O_2 saturation of hemoglobin by about 6%. Recalling that 98% or more of the blood O_2 is carried by hemoglobin, this 6% is sizeable. The Bohr relationship is especially valuable in the capillaries of exercising muscles, in the myocardium, and in the maternal/fetal exchange vessels of the placenta. In pathological situations as well, where fever elevates body temperature, then O_2 will be unloaded everywhere with greater ease. Shifting of the position of the oxyhemoglobin curve ensures O_2 delivery at the highest possible partial pressure.

D. THE CONCEPT OF P_{50}

Examination of *Figures 9-7* and *9-8* illustrate how an increase of blood CO_2 (or H^+) and body temperature can change the position of the oxyhemoglobin dissociation curve. It is easily seen that the middle portion of the curve is displaced the greatest amount. Thus, the most sensitive indicator of a curve shift to the left or right would be measurement of the PO_2 at 50% hemoglobin saturation. The term P_{50} thus refers to the PO_2 at which hemoglobin is half saturated.

The usual P_{50} seen in healthy arterial blood is 26 mmHg (3.5 kPa). In *Figure 9-8*, a 5°C rise in temperature, from 38°C to 43°C, increased the P_{50} from 26 mm Hg (3.5 kPa) to 34 mmHg (4.5 kPa). This rise occurred even though PCO_2 was maintained at a normal 40 mmHg (5.3 kPa), and resulted from an increasing acidity associated with an elevated body metabolism.

Hemoglobin is not necessarily restricted to the animal kingdom. Legumes such as peas and beans possess root nodules that play a role in N_2 fixation with the help of a substance called leghemoglobin. Its dissociation curve with O_2 is shifted even more to the left than that of myoglobin or HbF. Its P_{50} is only 0.04 mmHg (0.005 kPa), which increases the driving influx for O_2 into the root nodules by a factor of 10,000 times when compared to the driving influx of O_2 into the blood of adult humans.

E. THE ROLE OF 2,3-DPG IN OXYGEN DISSOCIATION

Because there are no mitochondria in erythrocytes, these cells have no Krebs cycle enzymes or cytochrome enzymes to unlock the vast quantities of energy residing in complete glucose metabolism to CO_2 and water. Instead, incomplete metabolism occurs, and glycolytic enzymes convert glucose to pyruvic acid. This diffuses into the plasma.

One of the intermediate compounds in this breakdown sequence is 1,3-diphosphoglyceric acid (1,3-DPG). Tissues other than erythrocytes convert this enzymatically to 3-phosphoglyceric acid and form one mole of ATP in the process. Erythrocytes, however, have an additional enzyme, 2,3-DPG mutase, which can convert 1,3-DPG to 2,3-DPG. This molecule does not diffuse across the erythrocyte cell membrane into the plasma, and instead either partially dissociates into H^+ ions and DPG^- ions, or, as shown in *Figure 9-9*, 2,3-DPG can be converted to 3-phosphoglyceric acid by another enzyme, 2,3-DPG phosphatase. Thus, 2,3-DPG is the pivotal molecule in a biochemical shunt (named to honor its discovers—the Rapoport-Luebering shunt) that serves as an alternative metabolic pathway in anaerobic metabolism.

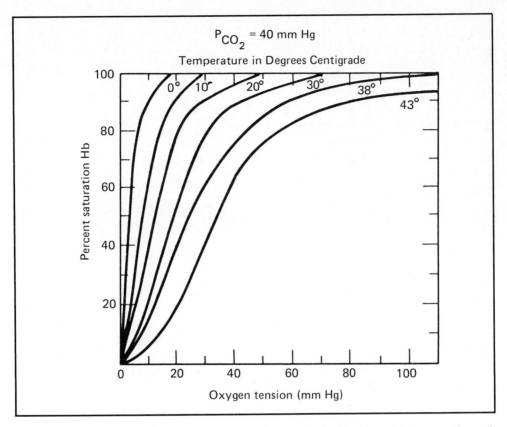

Figure 9-8. When body temperature is elevated, metabolism is increased, with a resulting increase in circulating blood metabolic acids, particularly lactic acid. Thus, even if the PCO_2 is kept constant at 40 mm Hg, the oxyhemoglobin curve shifts to the right with increasing acidity. This is explained by the heterotropic interaction between O_2 and H^+ when binding to hemoglobin. Commonly, the point on the curve where hemoglobin is 50% saturated with O_2—the P_{50} point—is considered when such changes are quantitated. A 5°C rise in temperature, from 38°C to 43°C, increases the P_{50} from 26 mm Hg (3.5 kPa) to 34 mm Hg (4.5 kPa).

The main acid-soluble constituent of erythrocytes in most mammals is 2,3-DPG—about 10 times greater than inorganic phosphate and 4 times greater than ATP. This is unique, for in other tissues it occurs only in trace amounts. When erythrocytes are stored under acid conditions, as in blood bank bags, the 2,3-DPG concentration decreases more rapidly than ATP, suggesting that it can function as a reservoir for ATP formation.

Hypoxia increases the proportion of reduced (deoxygenated) hemoglobin in the venous blood. Reduced hemoglobin has a specific and stoichiometric reaction with 2,3-DPG such that one mole of hemoglobin tetramer combines with one mole of 2,3-DPG ester to form a chemical complex. The deoxyhemoglobin/DPG complex is highly resistant to oxygenation; the DPG must be displaced in order

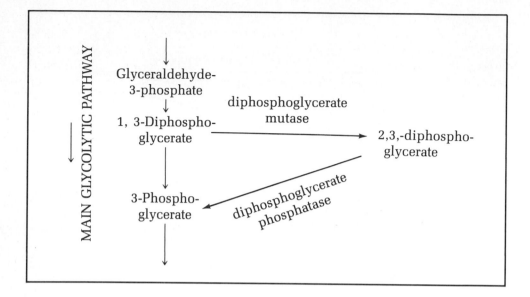

Figure 9-9. Diagram of the metabolic pathway by which certain quantities of glucose can be shunted into the formation of 2,3-diphosphoglyceric acid (2,3-DPG) in red blood cells instead of proceeding directly down its normal metabolic pathway to pyruvic acid. DPG is one of three ligands (the others being CO_2 and H^+) which lower the binding affinity of O_2 to hemoglobin.

for O_2 to bind. This complexing reduces the free diphosphoglycerate (DPG^-) ion concentration within the erythrocytes. Since 2,3-DPG has a rate-limiting function for both the glycolytic and the Rapoport-Luebering pathways, binding of it to hemoglobin increases the activity of these reactions.

The 2,3-DPG mechanism is one of three major processes governing tissue O_2 exchange. All have different time dimensions. 2,3-DPG time dynamics are measured in hours as it works to counter reductions in capillary or venous O_2 tension by increasing O_2 availability. It is intermediate in its time dynamics between the other two processes, the erythropoietin system, which requires weeks, and reflex blood flow changes that can occur within seconds.

An increase in blood pH of 0.01 unit, within the range of 7.30 to 7.50, will increase the erythrocyte DPG^- concentration by 5%, which is sufficient to increase the P_{50} by 1 mmHg (0.13 kPa). This relationship between the effects of pH on the O_2 affinity for hemoglobin and the self-regulating adjustment of the O_2 release to the tissues may be one explanation for the maintenance of plasma and erythrocyte pH in the living organism within such narrow limits. The DPG^- ion binds to the β chains of hemoglobin, and thus serves as a third important ligand (together with CO_2 and H^+ ions) that decreases O_2 affinity for hemoglobin. Its discovery was relatively recent, in 1967, simultaneously by two groups of investigators, Ruth and Reinhold Benesch, and Chanutin and Curnish.

Hemoglobin F (fetal) contains no β chains, and is unaffected by 2,3-DPG. This explains why the fetal oxyhemoglobin dissociation curve is displaced farther to the left of that for adult hemoglobin (Figure 9-6). In the uterine environment the arterial PO_2 is always low (but adequate), and hemoglobin F can quite efficiently meet the O_2 requirements of the fetus. Hemoglobin F is another excellent example of the concept that evolution has provided many subtle forms of the same basic molecule, each with properties to help serve differing gas transport requirements. Maternal arterial blood must transfer O_2 to the fetus via placental exchange with fetal blood. Thus, the fetal hemoglobin affinity for O_2 should be great enough that, when exposed to maternal blood, O_2 will cascade onto it. As maternal hemoglobin desaturates, fetal hemoglobin should become more saturated. This could occur only if the oxyhemoglobin saturation curve of hemoglobin F were shifted substantially to the left of that for HbA_1 or HbA_2. Work done with sheep has conclusively demonstrated this. Although the PO_2 of fetal umbilical vein blood is lower than that in the maternal uterine artery, the fetal hemoglobin concentration is higher. The end result is actually a higher circulating O_2 content in the fetus than in the mother.

TRANSPORT OF CARBON DIOXIDE IN THE BLOOD

A. MODES OF TRANSPORT

Inspired air contains insignificant amounts (0.04%) of CO_2. Unless it has been added to inspired gas, the CO_2 of venous blood, alveolar gas, and arterial blood originates with tissue metabolism. Each minute the metabolizing cells consume approximately 250 ml of O_2 and produce approximately 200 ml of CO_2. This permits calculation of a *respiratory exchange ratio* (R) of $CO_2/O_2 = 200/250 = 0.8$.

CO_2 is carried in plasma in a quantity about twice that found in the erythrocytes (Figure 9-10). Thus, if we consider a liter of mixed venous blood, 550 ml of plasma will contain 34.4 ml of CO_2 per 100 ml whereas 450 ml of erythrocytes will carry 18.6 ml/100 ml. If the sample were arterial blood, these values would be 32.6 ml/100 ml for plasma and 16.4 ml/100 ml for erythrocytes. Mixed venous blood contains about 7.6% more CO_2 than arterial blood.

CO_2 can be carried either in physical solution (dissolved PCO_2) or chemically bound (hydrated to form H_2CO_3 or combined with plasma proteins and hemoglobin). A CO_2 dissociation curve for whole blood can be produced by plotting blood CO_2 content as a function of changing PCO_2 (Figure 9-11). At low PCO_2 values, the slope of the curve is quite steep, but at PCO_2 values found commonly in the blood there is no tendency for the curve to plateau even though the slope decreases significantly. The implication of this slope is that it would be difficult to saturate the blood with CO_2 under ordinary conditions.

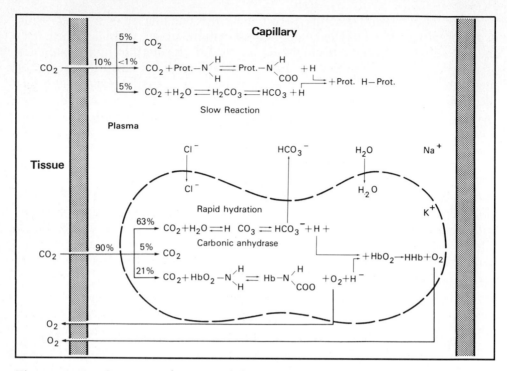

Figure 9-10. Summary diagram of the various fates of CO_2 as it diffuses from cells and interstitial space into the peripheral capillaries prior to its transport toward the venous circulation.

Hemoglobin is the principal binding site for CO_2 in erythrocytes, specifically to amino groups on the globin chains. The amino groups involved are the four α-NH_2 groups on the valine residues at the termini of the four peptide chains. Plasma proteins serve a similar role outside the erythrocytes, and the following describes the reaction:

$$Pr\text{-}NH_2 + CO_2 \rightleftharpoons Pr\text{-}NHCOO^- + H^+$$

Using Henry's law (Chapter Eight), it is possible to calculate the dissolved CO_2 in 100 ml of arterial and mixed venous blood. We can assume a P_aCO_2 of 40 mmHg (5.3 kPa) and a $P_{\bar{v}}CO_2$ of 47 mmHg (6.3 kPa). The dissolved CO_2 in arterial blood is then given by $P_aCO_2 = 0.067 \times 40 = 2.7$ ml/100 ml. The CO_2 in mixed venous blood is given by $P_{\bar{v}}CO_2 = 0.067 \times 47 = 3.1$ ml/100 ml. The P_aCO_2 is thus $2.7/0.30 = 9$ times greater than the P_aO_2. The P_aCO_2 is an even larger $3.1/0.12 = 26$ times greater than the $P_{\bar{v}}O_2$.

In arterial blood, the total CO_2 (dissolved plus bound) amounts to 49 ml/100 ml. In mixed venous blood this is 53 ml/100 ml. From the foregoing values for dissolved CO_2, it can be seen that in arterial blood, this accounts for $(2.7/49) \times 100 = 5.9\%$ of the total, leaving 94.1% in bound forms such as HCO_3^-, H_2CO_3, or carbamino compounds. In mixed venous blood, the dissolved CO_2 amounts to $(3.2/53) \times 100 = 6.0\%$, with 94% transported in the various bound forms.

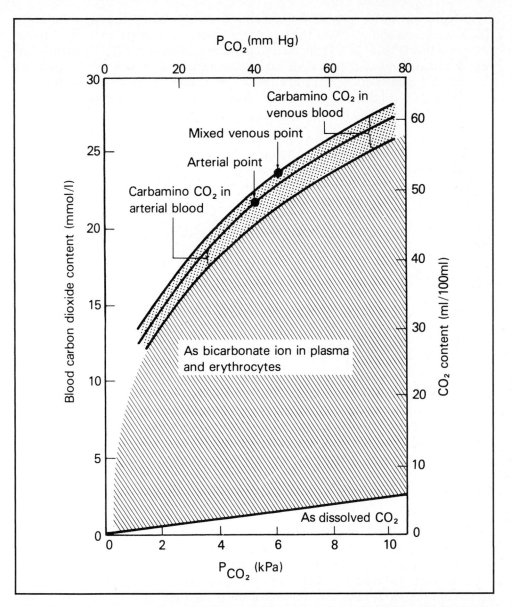

Figure 9-11. Carbon dioxide dissociation curve for whole blood. As PCO_2 rises, the quantities of dissolved CO_2 and HCO_3^- rise dramatically, and are relatively unaffected by the oxygenation state of hemoglobin. In contrast, the transport of CO_2 in the carbamino form is little influenced by the PCO_2, but significantly altered by the oxygenation status of hemoglobin. (Reprinted with permission from *Applied Respiratory Physiology*, by J.F. Nunn, 2nd ed., p. 341, Butterworths: London, 1977.)

Actually, the entire body serves as a large reservoir for storing CO_2. The body fluids represent about 70% of the body mass, and can average 50 ml of CO_2 per 100 ml of fluid. Thus, a 70 kg man contains about 35 liters of CO_2. Hyperventilation depletes some of these stores, and hypoventilation allows their accumulation. Bone contains more than 100 ml of CO_2 per 100 ml of tissue. During normal breathing, CO_2 production equals output according to the following equation:

$$\dot{V}CO_2 = F_ECO_2 \times \dot{V}_E.$$

Figure 9-10 illustrates the several transport forms of CO_2 as it moves either into the plasma or the erythrocytes. Although 90% of the gas enters the erythrocytes, in either these cells or in plasma the primary fate of CO_2 is hydration to form carbonic acid, with subsequent dissociation according to the equation:

$$H_2O + CO_2 \rightleftharpoons H_2CO_3 \rightleftharpoons H^+ + HCO_3^-$$

The reason for so much CO_2 entering the erythrocyte is explained by the presence of a zinc-containing enzyme, carbonic anhydrase, which enormously accelerates the hydration reaction. Recent studies using both bovine and human carbonic anhydrase suggest a catalytic effect as great as a millionfold at 25°C and pH = 7.0. The enzyme has 260 amino acids arranged in a chain, but shaped like a $4.1 \times 4.1 \times 4.7$ nm ellipsoid. The zinc ion is inside a 1.5 nm deep cavity, around which water molecules are oriented.

Carbonic anhydrase is present only in erythrocytes, certain kidney cells, pancreatic cells, and gastric mucosal cells. In each cell it helps to accelerate production of H_2CO_3 for generating of hydrogen ions (as in the gastric mucosal cells, for digestion) or bicarbonate ions (as in pancreatic cells, for pancreatic juice). The enzyme does not affect the ionic dissociation aspect, which already proceeds very fast. To indicate the relative concentrations of each of the components of the hydration equation for carbonic anhydrase, the equation can be expressed as follows, with numerical values in moles per liter $\times 10^{-8}$:

$$H_2O + CO_2 \rightleftharpoons H_2CO_3 \rightleftharpoons H^+ + HCO_3^-$$
$$120,000 \qquad 240 \qquad 4 \qquad 2,400,000$$

When carbonic acid dissociates, the products of the reaction, H^+ and HCO_3^-, do not accumulate in the erythrocytes. Many of the hydrogen ions bind to hemoglobin (to the globin chains) as well as with other buffers, releasing a potassium ion in exchange. This maintains the pH within the erythrocyte within 0.2 pH unit from the plasma. The equation is as follows:

$$H^+ + HCO_3^- + K^+ + Hb^- \rightarrow HHb + K^+ + HCO_3^-$$

Although HCO_3^- ions remain, the erythrocyte membrane is permeable to them, and they enter the plasma. Because the plasma membrane is only slightly permeable to cations such as Na^+ and K^+, the HCO_3^- departs unaccompanied by them. To eliminate any electropositivity from occurring within the erythrocyte, chloride ions from the plasma enter the cell by diffusion. This ion exchange is often termed the chloride-bicarbonate shift, and was first described by Hartog Hamburger, a Dutch physiologist.

B. EFFECTS OF OXYGEN ON HEMOGLOBIN-CO$_2$ INTERACTION

Recall that Bohr and co-workers described in 1904 the relationship whereby an increase in the PCO$_2$ of circulating blood, given a fixed PO$_2$, decreased the amount of O$_2$ carried by the blood. One would logically assume that the opposite should also be true. That is, if the PCO$_2$ is maintained constant, then if the PO$_2$ is increased, the amount of CO$_2$ that can be carried will decrease. Bohr spent the remaining 7 years of his life attempting to prove this, but failed. It remained for the Scottish physiologist at Oxford, John Scott Haldane, together with his colleague Charles Douglas and a young Danish woman scientist, Joanne Christiansen, to indeed demonstrate it, using Haldane's own blood, in 1914.

Thus, in peripheral tissues the Bohr effect is dominant, and O$_2$ tends to move into the tissues in part through the influence of metabolic CO$_2$. In the lungs, the Haldane effect dominates, with CO$_2$ tending to move into the alveoli in part through the influence of incoming atmospheric O$_2$.

The Haldane effect is graphed in *Figure 9–11*. When reduced hemoglobin (deoxyhemoglobin) and oxyhemoglobin are exposed to varying PCO$_2$ levels, their abilities to bind CO$_2$ are different. Reduced hemoglobin can carry more. The usually encountered CO$_2$ and P$_a$CO$_2$ values for arterial and venous blood are indicated in that figure by small letters a and v, respectively. The analogous relationship for the Bohr effect is graphed in *Figure 9–7*, with hemoglobin saturation with O$_2$ being plotted as a function of different PO$_2$ values. By observing the usually encountered values for arterial (a) and venous (v) blood, it can be seen that, the CO$_2$ dissociation curve is almost linear at body conditions, whereas the O$_2$ dissociation curve is markedly sigmoid in its shape. Thus, increases in PCO$_2$ bring about proportionate increases in the blood CO$_2$ content. Decreases in PO$_2$ can be marked without affecting O$_2$ content significantly.

The importance of carbonic anhydrase is seen when CO$_2$ is unloaded from the blood to the alveoli in the lungs. Without this enzyme, about 200 seconds would be required for the same amount of CO$_2$ to cross the alveolocapillary membrane. With transit time limited during resting conditions to 0.75 sec, and less with exercise, clearly this preservation of a CO$_2$ movement gradient via carbonic anhydrase is crucial.

RELEVANT READING

Astrand, I., Astrand, P-O, Christensen, E.H., and Hedman, R. Myoglobin as an oxygen store in man. *Acta Physiologica Scandinavica* **48**:454–460, 1960.

Ayres, S.M. Hemoglobin, evolution, and carbon monoxide. *Respiratory Care* **17**:291–294, 1972.

Bellingham, A.J., and Huehns, E.R. Compensation in haemolytic anemias caused by abnormal hemoglobins. *Nature* **218**:924–926, 1968.

Benesch, R., Benesch, R.E., and Enoki, Y. The interaction of hemoglobin and its subunits with 2, 3-diphosphoglycerate. *Proceedings of the National Academy of Sciences USA* **59**:526–532, 1968.

Bohr, C., Hasselbalch, K.A., and Krogh, A. Ueber einen in biologischer Beziehung wichtigen Einfluss, den die Kohlensaurespannung des Blutes auf dessen Sauerstoffbindung ubt. *Scandinavian Archives of Physiology* **16**:402–412, 1904.

Braasch, D. Red cell deformability and capillary blood flow. *Physiological Reviews* **51**:679–701, 1971.

Branemark, P.I., and Lindstrom, J. Shape of circulating blood corpuscles. *Biorheology* **1**:139–142, 1963.

Brewer, G.J., and Eaton, J.W. Erythrocyte metabolism: interaction with oxygen transport. *Science* **171**:1205–1211, 1971.

Brinkman, R., and Jouxis, J.H.P. The occurrence of several kinds of haemoglobin in human blood. *Journal of Physiology* (London) **85**:117–127, 1935.

Chanutin, A., and Curnish, R.R. Effect of organic and inorganic phosphates on the O_2 equilibrium of human erythrocytes. *Archives of Biochemistry* **121**:96–, 1967.

Desforges, J.F. Hemoglobin—a working molecule. *New England Journal of Medicine* **295**:164–165, 1976.

Douglas, C.G., Haldane, J.S., and Haldane, J.B.S. The laws of combination of hemoglobin with carbon monoxide and oxygen. *Journal of Physiology* **44**:275–304, 1912.

Edsall, J.T. Hemoglobin and the origins of allosterism. *Federation Proceedings* **39**:226–235, 1980.

Eichner, E.R. Sickle cell trait, exercise, and altitude. *Physician and Sports medicine* 14(11):144–157, 1986.

Haldane, J.S. The action of carbonic oxide on man. *Journal of Physiology* **18**:430–, 1895.

Harkness, D.R. The regulation of hemoglobin oxygenation. *Advances in Internal Medicine* **17**:189–214, 1971.

Hlastala, M.P., Standaert, T.A., Franada, R.L., and McKenna, H.P. Hemoglobin—ligand interaction in fetal and maternal sheep blood. *Respiration Physiology* **34**:185–194, 1978.

Holeton, G.F. Oxygen uptake and circulation by a hemoglobinless Antarctic fish (*Chaenocephalus aceratus* Lonnberg) compared with three red-blooded Antarctic fish. *Comparative Biochemistry and Physiology* **34**:457–471, 1970.

Kao, F.F. Gas transport functions of the blood. Chapter VI. *An Introduction to Respiratory Physiology*, Exerpta Medica, Amsterdam, pp. 105–126, 1979.

Kazazian, H.H., Jr., and Woodhead, A.P. Hemoglobin A synthesis in the developing fetus. *New England Journal of Medicine* **289**:58–62, 1973.

Lenfant, C., Torrance, J.D., Woodson, A.D., Jacobs, P., and Finch, C.A. Role of organic phosphates in the adaptation of man to hypoxia. *Federation Proceedings* **29**:1115–1117, 1970.

Lenfant, C., and Sullivan, K. Adaptation to high altitude. *New England Journal of Medicine* **284**:1298–1309, 1971.

Oelshlegl, F.J., Jr., Brewer, G.J., and Noble, N.A. Red cell 2,3-diphosphoglycerate differences between American Negroes and Caucasians. *IRCS Medical Sciences* **4**:497, 1976.

Perutz, M.F. The hemoglobin molecule. *Scientific American* **211**(5): 64–76, 1964.

Perutz, M.F. Stereochemistry of cooperative effects in haemoglobin. Haem-haem interaction and the problem of allostery. The Bohr effect and combination with organic phosphates. *Nature* **228**:726–733, 1970.

Perutz, M.F. Haemoglobin: the molecular lung. *New Scientist and Science Journal* **50**:676–679, 1971.

Perutz, M.F. Hemoglobin structure and respiratory transport. *Scientific American* **239**(6):92–123, 1978.

Pierson, D.J. The evolution of breathing: 5. Oxygen-carrying pigments: respiratory mass transit. *Respiratory Care* **27**:963–970, 1982.

Rapoport, S., and Luebering, J. Glycerate-2,3-diphosphatase. *Journal of Biological Chemistry* **189**:683–694, 1951.

Romero-Herrera, A.E., Lehmann, and H. Joysey, K.A. Molecular evolution of myoglobin and the fossil record: a phylogenetic synthesis. *Nature* **246**:389–395, 1973.

Rose, Z. Enzymes controlling 2,3-diphosphoglycerate in human erythrocytes. *Federation Proceedings* **29**:1105–1111, 1970.

Ruud, J.T. The ice fish. *Scientific American* **213**(5):108–114, 1965.

Skalak, R., and Branemark, P.J. Deformation of red blood cells in capillaries. *Science* **164**:717–719, 1969.

Steen, J.B., and Berg, T. The gills of two species of haemoglobin-free fishes compared to those of other teleosts—with a note on severe anemia in an eel. *Comparative Biochemistry and Physiology* **18**:517–526, 1966.

Vegas, A.M. Importance of oxygen transport in clinical medicine. *Critical Care Medicine* **7**:419–423, 1979.

Winterhalter, K.M. Does hemoglobin breathe, and if yes, how?—the T and R state of hemoglobin. *New England Journal of Medicine* **289**:41–42, 1973.

Woodson, R.D. O_2 transport: DPG and P_{50}. *Basics of RD* **5**(4):1–6, 1977.

Woodson, R.D. Physiological significance of oxygen dissociation curve shifts. *Critical Care Medicine* **7**:368–373, 1979.

Ventilatory Aspects of Acid-Base Problems

Chapter Ten

Chapter Ten Outline

General Principles Concerning Acid Production and Buffering

The Relationship Among CO_2, H^+, and H_2CO_3

Assessing Acid-Base Status

    A. Collecting a Blood Specimen for Analysis

    B. Interrelationship Between Blood pH and Ventilatory Status

    C. Assessment of Blood Bicarbonate and Base Excess

Acid-Base Derangements and Physiologic Compensation

    A. General Concepts

    B. Alveolar Hyperventilation with pH Variations
       Acute alveolar hyperventilation
       Chronic alveolar hyperventilation
       Examples of respiratory alkalosis
       Completely compensated metabolic acidosis
       Partially compensated metabolic acidosis
       Examples of metabolic acidosis

    C. Acceptable Alveolar Ventilation with pH Variations
       Metabolic alkalosis
       Metabolic acidosis

    D. Ventilatory Failure with pH variations
       Partially compensated metabolic alkalosis
       Chronic ventilatory failure
       Acute ventilatory failure
       Examples of respiratory acidosis

Assessing Oxygenation Status in the Context of Acid-Base Regulation

    A. Arterial PO_2

    B. Hemoglobin-Oxygen Affinity

    C. Blood O_2 Content

Metabolism of body fuels—carbohydrates and fatty acids and sometimes protein—results in their complete oxidation to CO_2, H_2O and free energy. If insufficient O_2 is available, carbohydrates may be metabolized temporarily to intermediates such as pyruvic and lactic acid, with much less free energy available for producing movement and heat. The majority of the CO_2 is hydrated to carbonic acid (H_2CO_3), with resulting dissociation into hydrogen (H^+) and bicarbonate (HCO_3^-) ions. Lactic and pyruvic acids similarly dissociate into pyruvate$^-$ or lactate$^-$ ions and H^+ ions. This constant infusion of H^+ ions into the body fluids as a result of ongoing metabolism can pose some significant problems if the accumulation is too great or if removal is inadequate. The vast majority of biochemical synthetic and degradative reactions in the body are enzymatically controlled. Enzymes are designed to function only within a very narrow range of hydrogen ion concentration $[H^+]$. Thus, means must be available to preserve this ionic equilibrium. In addition to their crucial role in regulating enzymatic reactions, H^+ ions are powerful vasodilators and strong stimulants of ventilation. Maintenance of normal circulatory and ventilatory dynamics also requires a constant regulation of $[H^+]$.

Three major organ systems devote much of their activity toward regulating acid and alkali levels: the lungs, the blood, and the kidneys. Buffering of metabolic acids is carried out largely by the blood and kidneys, whereas excretion of acids is handled by the lungs and kidneys. Metabolism produces about 12,000 milliequivalents (mEq) of H^+ per day, and 99% of this is excreted by the lungs as CO_2. CO_2 is the body's most important acid. It is a volatile acid because of its gaseous nature, compared to non-volatile acids, such as lactic acid (from anaerobic glycolysis), ketoacids (produced by fatty acid metabolism), and other organic acids (notably those absorbed through digestion—one example would be the salicylic acid in aspirin). The kidneys also play a role in H^+ ion excretion, working precisely, and their role in buffering acidity is probably as important as in excreting acid or retaining HCO_3^-.

The importance of the lungs in acid-base regulation is easy to understand. Ventilatory failure increases the $[H^+]$ in arterial blood, resulting in respiratory acidosis. Similarly, alveolar hyperventilation can decrease the $[H^+]$ in arterial blood, causing respiratory alkalosis. The time-related changes in ventilatory and renal function are quite different. Within minutes after the cessation of breathing, acid-base problems can be life-threatening. With renal shutdown, this will not occur for several days. This Chapter discusses some of these fascinating relationships as they affect organ system function in the body.

GENERAL PRINCIPLES CONCERNING ACID PRODUCTION AND BUFFERING

Free H^+ ions are rare in most body fluids. It would require 25 million liters of body fluid to yield just one gram of H^+ ions in arterial blood. Pure H_2O has considerably more—it would only take 10 million liters to yield one gram of H^+ ions. It is unwieldy to express H^+ ion concentrations as 1×10^{-7} moles/L (the $[H^+]$ in pure H_2O) or 4×10^{-8} mole/L (the $[H^+]$ in arterial blood). A better terminology is appropriate. Sorenson in 1909 proposed usage of the small letter p as the "hydrogen ion exponent." Then the term "pH" represents the negative logarithm of the $[H^+]$. Thus, $pH = -\log_{10}[H^+]$. For H_2O, $pH = -\log_{10}$ of 1×10^{-7} $= 7$. Note that the logarithmic nature of the scale is such that a solution with $pH = 6$ is 10 times more acidic than a solution with $pH = 7$, and a solution with $pH = 5$ is 100 times more acidic. Many of today's cola drinks, with their carbonation, and their pH of about 3.0, are thus 10,000 times more acidic than pure water. A decrease of 0.3 pH unit represents a doubling of the $[H^+]$.

During the 1960s Poul Astrup recommended that SI units be used instead of pH units for quantifying H^+ ions in solution. The appropriate unit would be nanomoles/L, where 1×10^{-7} mole/L $= 100 \times 10^{-9}$ mole/L $= 100$ nanomoles/ L. The relationship of pH units and nanomoles/L for the blood acidity variations found in life is summarized in Table 10-1. The range of normal values in most clinical laboratories is 35 to 42 nanomoles/L ($pH = 7.45$ to 7.38).

When metabolic acids enter the venous blood, that blood resists the change in its acidity. This is because there are buffering substances in that blood which act to minimize the pH change. It is essential that such substances exist. A deviation of 0.5 arterial pH unit from the normal value of 7.42 in man can be dangerous to health. Each day the body accumulates almost 100 liters of 0.1 N acid which gets eliminated in the form of CO_2. There indeed had better be some effective mechanisms for handling all this acid! Along with ingestion of acids, alkaline substances are also taken in through the diet. Altered metabolism during certain disease states can produce additional quantities of acid. Despite all this, arterial and venous blood pH remain remarkably constant in health, thanks to powerfully effective systems for excreting acid, retaining base, and buffering both.

A buffer solution is a weak acid (such as H_2CO_3) or base plus a salt (such as $NaHCO_3$) of that weak acid or base. Weakness implies minimum dissociation of the acid or base into its component ionic species. A common buffer solution in blood is a mixture of $NaHCO_3$ and H_2CO_3, with primarily the $NaHCO_3$ dissociated. Addition of more H^+ (as CO_2 moves from tissue cells into the blood) results in more H_2CO_3 being formed, thereby tying up many H^+ ions and minimizing a pH change. Another important buffer is the hemoglobin molecule.

THE RELATIONSHIP AMONG CO_2, H^+, AND H_2CO_3

If we define an acid as any substance which increases $[H^+]$ or which donates a proton (a H^+ ion is a proton), then both CO_2 and H_2CO_3 are indeed acids, as a result of their dissociation in solution. During the ten years (1904–1914) between the written formulations of the Bohr and Haldane relationships (Chapter Nine)

TABLE 10-1. Conversion of H⁺ ion concentration to pH and nanomoles/liter.

pH	nanomoles of H^+/L	$[H^+]$ in moles/L
8.00	10.0	10.0×10^{-9}
7.95	11.2	11.2×10^{-9}
7.90	12.6	12.6×10^{-9}
7.85	14.1	14.1×10^{-9}
7.80	15.8	15.8×10^{-9}
7.75	17.8	17.8×10^{-9}
7.70	20.0	20.0×10^{-9}
7.65	22.4	22.4×10^{-9}
7.60	24.4	24.4×10^{-9}
7.55	28.2	28.2×10^{-9}
7.50	31.6	31.6×10^{-9}
7.45	35.5	35.5×10^{-9}
7.40	39.8	39.8×10^{-9}
7.35	44.6	44.6×10^{-9}
7.30	50.2	50.2×10^{-9}
7.25	56.3	56.3×10^{-9}
7.20	63.0	63.0×10^{-9}
7.15	71.0	71.0×10^{-9}
7.10	79.5	79.5×10^{-9}
7.05	89.0	89.0×10^{-9}
7.00	100.0	100.0×10^{-9}
6.95	112.0	112.0×10^{-9}
6.90	126.0	126.0×10^{-9}
6.85	141.0	141.0×10^{-9}
6.80	158.0	158.0×10^{-9}

the details of this dissociation were studied intensively by Lawrence J. Henderson.

Henderson's great interests in both physical and natural sciences led him to enter medical school at Harvard University in 1898. Graduating in 1902 cum laude, he then pursued research in laboratory clinical medicine at Cambridge, England, and began to work on a topic which had long interested him, namely the physiologic acid-base interrelationships between H_2CO_3 and $NaHCO_3$. In 1909, he reported on the relationships between dissolved CO_2, H_2CO_3, H^+, and HCO_3^-. He realized that the following equation was certainly true:

$$H_2O + CO_2 \rightleftharpoons H_2CO_3 \rightleftharpoons H^+ + HCO_3^-$$

But H_2CO_3 in the body is a rare and transitory intermediate between CO_2 and HCO_3^-. Hence he considered it more practical to treat CO_2 as the real proton donor rather than H_2CO_3.

It should be remembered that acids are classified according to the ease with which they give up their H^+ ions in forming a dissociative chemical equilibrium. Using HAc to represent any acid, then $HAc \rightleftharpoons H^+ + Ac^-$. A weak acid is one which does not readily dissociate. When it does, the anion (the negatively charged moiety) still has a rather strong affinity for H^+ and is characterized as a rather strong base. In low pH solutions, most weak acids are almost completely undissociated—as soon as they lose a H^+ ion, another replaces it. As the pH increases, this acid dissociates more and more. For any acid, there is a particular pH at which half of the acid will be dissociated and half undissociated. This pH is called the pK. It is the $-\log_{10}[H^+]$ at which 50% dissociation occurs. The higher the pK, the weaker the acid.

The pK of H_2CO_3 is about 3.4. At pH $= 7.4$, the ratio of HCO_3^- / H_2CO_3 is about 10,000 to 1. Since CO_2 is physiologically more useful in this context than H_2CO_3, being 500 times more abundant, Henderson approximated by assuming that it is CO_2 and not H_2CO_3 that is important, and used the ratio of HCO_3^- to CO_2. He then corrected the pK to account for the use of CO_2. This corrected or "approximated" pK equals 6.11. Thus, Henderson's now famous approximation equation of 1909 was the simple statement that:

$$[H^+] = K \times \frac{acid}{base} = K \times \frac{CO_2}{HCO_3^-}$$

It was in that same year that Sorenson's concept of pH emerged, and 7 years went by before the Danish physician Karl Hasselbalch took Henderson's equation and restated it in the context of this newer terminology. Hence, we now use the Hasselbalch form of the Henderson equation, stated simply as:

$$pH = pK + \log_{10} \frac{base}{acid} = pK + \log_{10} \frac{HCO_3^-}{CO_2}$$

This equation is of great significance in understanding acid-base equilibria in the body. First, it explains the behavior of the most abundant plasma buffer. Second, the pH and CO_2 can be measured by independent methods, and accurately, allowing calculation of HCO_3^-. Third, one can understand both the direction of an acid-base disturbance (by examining pH and noting the possibility of acidemia or alkalemia) and the source of the disturbance (CO_2 deviations imply respiratory malfunction, HCO_3^- deviations suggest metabolic problems).

Under healthy conditions one can measure HCO_3^- as 24 mEq per liter. For an anion such as HCO_3^-, with its oxidation state of -1, 24mM/L $= 24$ mEq/L. CO_2 is typically measured in mmHg or kPa. To permit meaningful assessment of CO_2 in relation to HCO_3^-, similar units must be used. Thus, CO_2 must be converted from mmHg to mEq/L. Recall from Chapter Eight that the solubility coefficient (α) for CO_2 in plasma $= 0.510$ ml/ml plasma $= 510$ ml/L plasma. It is also true that 22.6 ml $CO_2 = 1$mM $CO_2 = 1$ mEq CO_2. Thus, 1 ml $CO_2 = 0.044$ mM CO_2. Therefore,

$$\frac{510 \text{ ml/L/mm Hg} \times 0.044 \text{ mM } CO_2/ml}{760 \text{ mmHg}} = 0.03 \text{ m Eq/L} = 0.03 \text{ mM/L}$$

We also recall from Henry's law that the concentration of a gas in solution (C_G) is related to its partial pressure and its solubility. Thus, for CO_2, Cco_2 = PCO_2 × 0.03. If P_aCO_2 = 40 mmHg, then [CO_2] = 40 × 0.03 = 1.2 mEq/L. The total blood CO_2 will be presented by the sum of [HCO_3^-] and [CO_2], i.e., normally 24 mEq/L + (40 mmHg × 0.03 = 1.2 mEq/L) = 25.2 mEq/L. The ratio of HCO_3^- to CO_2 in healthy arterial blood is 24/1.2 = 20. The log_{10} of 20 = 1.3. Using the Henderson/ Hasselbalch equation to determine the pH of healthy arterial blood, we can then write:

$$pH = pK + log_{10} \frac{[HCO_3^-]}{[CO_2]} = 6.1 + 1.3 = 7.4$$

The ratio of 20:1 HCO_3^-/CO_2 is maintained partly by pulmonary ventilation and partly by metabolism. The ventilatory aspect is summarized below:

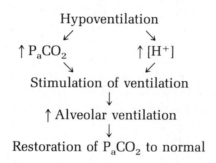

This delicate mechanism operates only when: (1) the sensitivity of the respiratory center is normal; (2) the nervous connections between the respiratory center and the ventilatory muscles are intact; (3) the ventilatory muscles are completely functional; and (4) the lung is not seriously diseased.

ASSESSING ACID-BASE STATUS

A. COLLECTING A BLOOD SPECIMEN FOR ANALYSIS

To properly understand O_2/CO_2 dynamics in active tissues requires assessment of ventilation, oxygenation, and acid-base variables together. Arterial blood gas analysis has become a vital tool in pulmonary medicine for the assessment of all these variables. Arterial blood is more useful to study than venous blood. Blood obtained from a vein gives information primarily about the region perfused by that blood. Depending upon the site of collection, information obtained from venous blood can be quite misleading about the metabolism of the body as a whole, and will provide a poor indication of what the lungs have done to make the blood fit for transport to the heart and other body tissues. It could be said that in this instance we are more interested in the future of the patient (where all of the blood is going) than in the patient's past (where some of the blood has been), although of course the past will modify the future somewhat.

The radial artery is preferred for routine sampling, with brachial and femoral arteries as good alternates. The dead space of the needle and the syringe are heparinized. The sample should not be exposed to air because P_aCO_2 will fall and P_aO_2 will rise. The sample should be analyzed immediately or else placed on ice to decrease erythrocyte metabolism. At 37°C the pH will fall by 0.06 units per hour, the P_aO_2 will fall by 3 to 12 mm Hg per hour (0.4 to 1.6 kPa/hr), and the P_aCO_2 will rise by 5 mmHg per hour (0.7 kPa/hr). In the laboratory the blood sample is injected into the chamber of an instrument with electrodes constructed to allow measurement of PO_2, PCO_2, and pH.

The Severinghaus electrode is a glass pH electrode surrounded by an unchanging buffer solution; this is separated from the blood sample by a plastic gas-permeable membrane. As blood CO_2 equilibrates with the solution, a pH change is measured by the glass electrode. The greater the CO_2 content, the greater the pH change. pH itself is determined using another electrode. The Clark electrode measures O_2. Here, blood PO_2 equilibrates with a solution in contact with a small platinum surface having a negative electrical charge. Oxygen molecules are broken down rapidly at the platinum surface, causing a change in ionic current that is measurable as a change in current flow between the silver electrode (anode) and the platinum electrode (cathode).

B. INTERRELATIONSHIP BETWEEN BLOOD pH AND VENTILATORY STATUS

The acid-base status is best assessed by consideration of arterial blood pH:

$$pH = 7.35 - 7.45 \Rightarrow \text{normal laboratory range}$$
$$pH > 7.45 \Rightarrow \text{alkalemia} \Rightarrow \uparrow HCO_3^- \text{ or } \downarrow P_aCO_2$$
$$pH < 7.35 \Rightarrow \text{acidemia} \Rightarrow \downarrow HCO_3^- \text{ or } \uparrow P_aCO_2$$

Ventilatory status is best assessed by measurement of dissolved CO_2 in the arterial blood:

$$P_aCO_2 = 35 \text{ to } 45 \text{ mmHg (4.7 to 6.0 kPa) is the normal laboratory range}$$
$$P_aCO_2 > 45 \text{ mmHg (6.0 kPa) implies ventilatory failure (alveolar}$$
$$\text{hypoventilation)}$$
$$P_aCO_2 < 35 \text{ mmHg (4.7 kPa) implies alveolar hyperventilation}$$

The pH and P_aCO_2 are obviously interrelated. CO_2 is an acid; an elevated P_aCO_2 increases the blood acidity. A condition of high P_aCO_2 and low pH represents respiratory acidosis. A low P_aCO_2 and high pH represents respiratory alkalosis.

Table 10-2 summarizes various values for arterial pH and PCO_2 that characterize both the normal healthy population and those individuals who are outside this normal population. It should be recalled that a range of one standard deviation above and below the mean represents 68% of the total values, whereas a range of two standard deviations represents 95% of the population. It is this group of values spanning two standard deviations that comprise the *laboratory normal population*. There is, however, 5% of the normal range outside this limit of two standard deviations. These values, although displaced considerably from the mean, are still seldom of therapeutic importance. This entire normal range is termed the *acceptable therapeutic range*. Thus, the laboratory normal range for P_aCO_2 is 35–45 mmHg (4.7–6.0 kPa), whereas the acceptable therapeutic range is 30–50 mmHg (4.0–6.7 kPa).

TABLE 10-2.   Terminology and Values for Arterial pH and PCO$_2$ Variations

	pH	P_aCO_2 mm Hg	P_aCO_2 kPa
Laboratory Normal Population Mean	7.40	40	5.3
± 1 standard deviation	7.38–7.42	38–42	5.1–5.6
± 2 standard deviations	7.53–7.45	35–45	4.7–6.0
Acceptable Normal Range	7.30–7.50	30–50	4.0–6.7
Values Outside Normal Range			
Alkalemia	>7.50		
Acidemia	<7.30		
Ventilatory failure		>50	>6.7
Alveolar hyperventilation		<30	<4.0

C. ASSESSMENT OF BLOOD BICARBONATE AND BASE EXCESS

Other important variables that need quantitation include HCO_3^- and an assessment of whether this HCO_3^- is in excess or in deficit. Bicarbonate is a value which is calculated from the arterial pH and PCO_2, using the Henderson-Hasselbalch equation. This, however, demands a readily functional knowledge of logarithms. In 1963 Ole Siggaard-Andersen published a nomographic relationship between pH, PCO_2, HCO_3^- and other variables, such that if two were known, then the others could be estimated simply by using a straight-edge ruler to extend a line connecting the two known points. Figure 10-1 reprints this nomogram from the original publication; since then it has appeared in many modified forms, and has greatly simplified the estimation of HCO_3^- once arterial pH and PCO_2 are determined.

The term *base excess* denotes the quantity of base (HCO_3^-, in mEq/L) that is above or below the normal range of buffer base in the body (22 to 28 mEq/L; mean

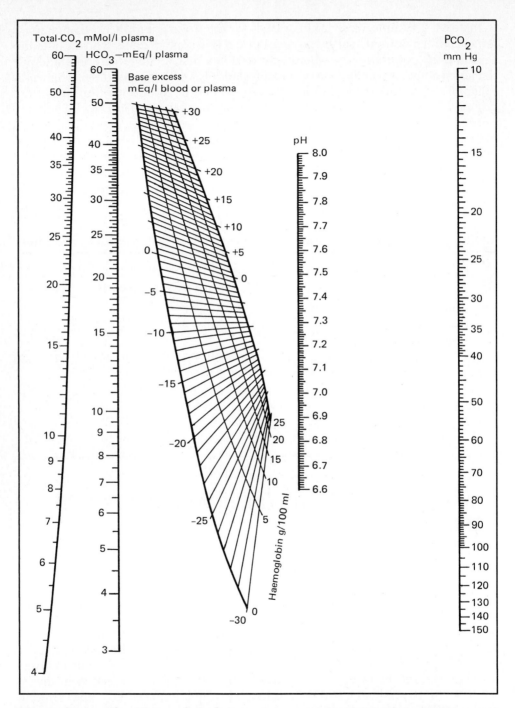

Figure 10-1. The Siggaard-Andersen nomogram for determining HCO_3^- and base excess. Reprinted with permission from Siggaard-Andersen, O. *Scandinavian Journal of Laboratory and Clinical Investigation* **15**:ff. 213, 1963.

= 24 mEq/L). Base excess cannot be determined solely by consideration of pH and P_aCO_2 because red blood cells are very important in buffering as well (see Chapter Nine). Thus, the hemoglobin level must also be considered. Using the Siggaard-Andersen nomogram, one can easily estimate the base excess by connecting three points: pH, P_aCO_2, and hemoglobin. Using that nomogram, as an example, an individual with a pH of 7.37, a P_aCO_2 of 23 mmHg (3.1 kPa), and a hemoglobin concentration of 15 gm/dl would have a base excess of -2 mEq/L. Thus, there is a slight shortage of buffer base. This negative base excess is also termed *base deficit*. Generally, a base deficit of less than 10 mEq/L is not considered sufficient for therapeutic treatment.

It is possible to estimate base excess or base deficit in another way if hemoglobin concentration is known to be normal. This technique was introduced by Barry Shapiro and is presented in his textbook *Clinical Interpretation of Arterial Blood Gases*. It is presented below in brief outline form. The calculations depend for their validity on two relationships. One is that, within physiologic limits, for each 20 mmHg (2.7 kPa) increase in the P_aCO_2 level above 40 mmHg (5.3 kPa), a concomitant decrease of 0.10 pH unit should occur. Thus, if a normal blood pH of 7.40 and a normal blood P_aCO_2 of 40 mmHg (5.3 kPa) are measured, then, if the P_aCO_2 rises to 60 mmHg (8 kPa), the blood pH will fall to 7.30. Similarly, for each 10 mmHg (1.4 kPa) fall in the P_aCO_2 level below 40 mmHg, an increase of 0.10 pH unit should occur. The other relationship is that a 10 mEq/L decrease in the available buffer base will decrease the pH by 0.15 unit.

Using these relationships to estimate base excess or deficit, the first step is to estimate the respiratory pH to identify the respiratory component of the clinical situation. From that, the base excess is easily determined. Consider the following example, where the pH is 7.24, the P_aCO_2 is 28 mmHg (3.8 kPa), and the Hb is 15 gm/dl.

(a) Find the difference between P_aCO_2 and 40 mmHg
40 mm Hg $-$ 28 mmHg $=$ 12 mmHg.

(b) Move the decimal two places to the left
12 becomes 0.12

(c_1) If the P_aCO_2 is $>$ 40 mmHg, subtract half the difference from 7.40 to estimate a predicted respiratory pH

(c_2) If the P_aCO_2 is $<$ 40 mmHg, add the entire difference to 7.40. Here
7.40 $+$ 0.12 $=$ 7.52

(d) Find the difference between the measured and predicted respiratory pH
7.24 $-$ 7.52 $=$ -0.28

(e) Move the decimal two places to the right
-0.28 becomes -28

(f) Multiply by 2/3 to calculate base excess
$-28 \times 2 = -56/3 = -18$ mEq/L

A graphic representation first published in 1948 by Horace Davenport has proved equally valuable in assessing acid-base relationships, especially as they change with time in any given individual. Since the Henderson-Hasselbalch equation relates the HCO_3^-, pH and P_aCO_2, these variables can be graphically expressed. *Figure 10-2* shows arterial HCO_3^- in mM/L plotted as a function of arterial pH.

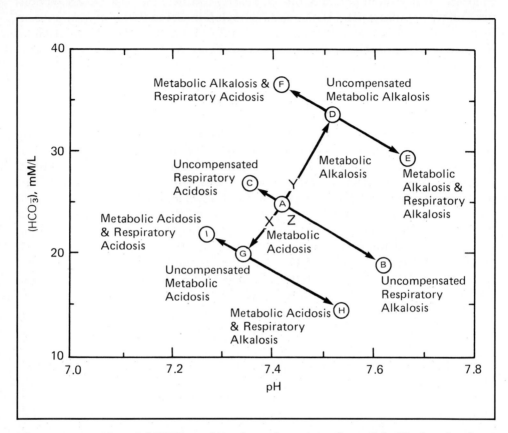

Figure 10-2.   Arterial HCO_3^- plotted as a function of arterial pH, showing how various kinds of acid-base derangements—both metabolic and respiratory in origin—can be characterized. Reprinted with permission from *The ABC of Acid-Base Chemistry*, by H. W. Davenport, 6th ed., p. 69, Univ. Chicago Press, 1974.

One can experimentally determine the pH of arterial blood to which various concentrations of HCO_3^- are added, all the while maintaining the P_aCO_2 constant at 40 mmHg (5.3 kPa). If these pH values are then plotted on the graph illustrated in *Figure 10-2*, a P_aCO_2 = 40 mmHg (5.3 kPa) isobar (line of constant pressure) is obtained. In this manner it becomes easy to characterize metabolic acidosis and alkalosis in terms of the HCO_3^- and pH changes they produce.

Consider the following example: the top finishers at a track meet in the 800 meter run as they cross the finish line. They will have incurred a sizable oxygen debt because ventilation would have been insufficient to allow them to run at nearly top speed and still bring in adequate oxygen for complete metabolism of body fuels. The P_aCO_2 will be unchanged from that measured during rest, but metabolic (lactic) acid levels in the venous and arterial blood will be elevated. The available blood HCO_3^- will partially buffer the lactic acid, leaving sodium lactate, a lowered blood HCO_3^- content, and somewhat decreased pH. On the $P_aCO_2 = 40$ mmHg (5.3 kPa) isobar, these athletes are now *(Figure 10-2)*, positioned below and to the left of the normal resting value, indicating metabolic acidosis (point X).

Now consider an individual who consumes a very heavy meal, typical of the traditional American Thanksgiving Day turkey dinner with all the trimmings. The gastric mucosa can concentrate H^+ ions one million times in comparison to plasma as it produces hydrochloric acid in preparation for digestion *(Figure 10-3)*. Particularly following a large meal, this H^+ ion sequestering into the gastric mucosa results in an increased conversion of blood CO_2 to HCO_3^- and H^+ ions. While the H^+ ions disappear from the blood, the elevated HCO_3^- results in metabolic alkalosis. This alkalosis is termed the postprandial alkaline tide. The P_aCO_2 remains at 40 mmHg (5.3 kPa), but the position of individuals on the pH-HCO_3^- plot would be a little above and to the right of normal resting values (Point Y on *Figure 10-2*).

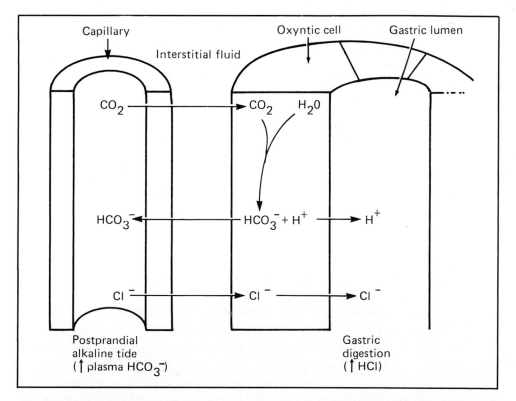

Figure 10-3. Diagram illustrating temporary post-prandial alkalinization of blood caused by oxyntic cell concentration of H^+ to permit gastric digestion.

Finally, consider an individual who is suffering from emotional hyperventilation—military parachutists about to take their first jump. As they are sitting in the airplane that will take them up to 2,500 feet (760 m) for their jump, their nervous jitters, coupled perhaps with the type of babbling small-talk often associated with anxiety states, can cause hyperventilation. Their P_aCO_2 will fall, their pH will rise, and their HCO_3^- level will fall. They will no longer be on the PCO_2 = 40 mmHg (5.3 kPa) isobar, and their respiratory alkalosis will position them appropriately on the HCO_3^- – plot in *Figure 10-2* (Point Z).

ACID-BASE DERANGEMENTS AND PHYSIOLOGIC COMPENSATION

A. GENERAL CONCEPTS

The normal homeostatic mechanisms of the body interact to compensate for respiratory and metabolic acid-base imbalances, with the lungs and kidneys acting largely in reciprocal fashion. Thus, in ventilatory disorders, the arterial blood pH is gradually returned to its normal range by renal retention or excretion of HCO_3^-. Similarly, in metabolic disorders, the lungs compensate by varying the P_aCO_2 levels through hypoventilation or hyperventilation, again attempting to normalize arterial blood pH. *Figure 10-4* summarizes these responses.

ACID BASE DISORDER	COMPENSATORY MECHANISM
Respiratory Acidosis ↑ P_aCO_2; ↓ pH	↑ retention of HCO_3^- by kidney to ↑ HCO_3^- and slowly ↑ pH
alveolar ventilation respiratory alkalosis ↓ P_aCO_2; ↑ pH	↑ excretion of HCO_3^- by kidney to ↓ HCO_3^- and gradually ↑ pH
metabolic acidosis ↓ HCO_3^-; ↓ pH	hyperventilation by lungs to ↓ P_aCO_2 and gradually ↑ pH
metabolic alkalosis ↑ HCO_3^-; ↑ pH	hypoventilation by lungs to ↑ P_aCO_2 and ↓ pH

Figure 10-4. Types of compensatory mechanisms occurring in chronic acid-base disorders. Remember that the kidneys provide compensation for respiratory acid-base problems, while the lungs provide compensation for metabolic acid-base disorders. The former acts through HCO_3^- regulation, the latter by CO_2 regulation.

Table 10-3 provides an outline for interpretation of arterial pH and PCO$_2$ values in acid-base derangements. Because CO$_2$ is the body's most important acid, it is useful to assess first and foremost the status of P$_a$CO$_2$. Then, one may attempt an interpretation of arterial blood pH values in the context of whether CO$_2$ is being retained or excreted (or kept within acceptable levels) as a result of a primarily ventilatory or metabolic problem.

B. ALVEOLAR HYPERVENTILATION WITH pH VARIATIONS

Acute alveolar hyperventilation (P$_a$CO$_2$ < 30 mmHg (4 kPa) and pH > 7.50. Because the arterial pH is unacceptably high, i.e., higher than the accepted range of 7.30 to 7.50, (Table 10-2), we can conclude that no renal compensation for the observed decrease in P$_a$CO$_2$ has occurred. Thus the P$_a$CO$_2$ change from its normal range must be relatively recent, so it is termed acute. The pH alteration is, therefore, secondary to the ventilatory change.

Chronic alveolar hyperventilation (P$_a$CO$_2$ < 30 mmHg (4 kPa) and pH 7.40 − 7.50. The acceptable arterial pH suggests that the kidneys are compensating for a chronic condition of decreased P$_a$CO$_2$ (from hyperventilation) by excreting HCO$_3^-$. The primary problem, therefore, is ventilatory and the compensation is adequate.

Examples of respiratory alkalosis. The two conditions described above are clear-cut instances of respiratory-induced alkalosis. It can occur from a variety of circumstances. Emotional derangements such as hallucinations or grief-induced anxiety states can bring temporary hyperventilation. Central nervous system diseases such as meningitis and encephalitis can increase the activity of brain stimulatory mechanisms for breathing (these will be discussed in Chapter Eleven). Hypoxia caused from temporary ascent to very high altitudes, especially above 10,000 ft (3,300 m) can stimulate breathing by activating peripheral breathing mechanisms (the aortic and carotid body chemoreceptors, which also will be discussed in Chapter Eleven).

Completely compensated metabolic acidosis (P$_a$CO$_2$ < 30 mmHg (4 kPa) and pH 7.35 to 7.45). One might logically consider this combination of pH and P$_a$CO$_2$ values as indicating alveolar hyperventilation with the kidneys a little overly active in their compensation, i.e., excreting so much HCO$_3^-$ that compensation is even on the acid side of the normal mean of 7.40. However, in fact, this logic is inappropriate, because one must always remember that, while compensation may in many instances not be adequate enough, overcompensation most probably will not occur. This is explained by the biological principle of symmorphosis (see Chapter One). Thus, another explanation is more appropriate. There is a primary metabolic problem, and the lungs are acting (successfully) to help return the blood pH to an acceptable range. There is thus a compensating respiratory alkalosis that is blowing off CO$_2$.

Partially compensated metabolic acidosis (P$_a$CO$_2$ < 30 mmHg (4 kPa) and pH < 7.30). Both P$_a$CO$_2$ and pH are profoundly changed (lowered) in this situation.

TABLE 10-3. Interpretation of Arterial pH and PCO$_2$ Values in Acid-Base Derangements

P$_a$CO$_2$ < 30 mmHg

pH < 7.30 Partially compensated metabolic acidosis	pH 7.30–7.40 Completely compensated metabolic acidosis	pH 7.40–7.50 Chronic alveolar hyperventilation	pH > 7.50 Acute alveolar hyperventilation

P$_a$CO$_2$ 30–50 mmHg

pH < 7.30 Metabolic acidosis	pH 7.30–7.50 Acceptable ventilatory and metabolic status	pH > 7.50 Metabolic alkalosis

P$_a$CO$_2$ > 50 mmHg

pH < 7.30 Acute ventilatory failure	pH 7.30–7.50 Chronic ventilatory failure	pH > 7.50 Partially compensated metabolic alkalosis

This indicates a distinct metabolic acidosis with even a vigorous alveolar hyperventilation inadequate to compensate for it.

Examples of metabolic acidosis. Metabolic acidosis can result either from an excessive production of H^+ ions or an excessive loss of HCO_3^-. The latter situation is best exemplified by chronic diarrhea. The former condition has at least three well-known examples. One involves circulatory shutdown, caused by lowered blood pressure or cardiac failure. Oxygen is not distributed adequately to supply the requirements of Krebs cycle conversion of pyruvic acid into CO_2, H_2O, and energy. Intermediate metabolites such as lactic acid accumulate, and acidosis results. Oftentimes, simply by improving the general oxygenation state of the patient, the patient's health status can be improved.

A second example includes starvation, diabetes mellitus, or a high fat diet, where carbohydrates are not available to the cells for metabolism. The cells compensate for this by instead mobilizing and metabolizing fatty acids. Krebs cycle activity declines, and acetyl coenzyme A is converted preferentially into acetoacetyl coenzyme A, and then into any of three substances collectively known as ketone bodies: acetoacetic acid, β-hydroxybutyric acid, and acetone. Two of these are non-volatile organic acids and contribute to metabolic acidosis. A diabetic patient hyperventilates to compensate for this metabolic acidosis. The hyperpnea and tachypnea form a characteristic respiratory pattern called Kussmaul's breathing, after the German physician, Adolph Kussmaul, who first described it.

A third example involves failure of kidney function to excrete H^+ ions. These ions accumulate, and in turn decrease the HCO_3^- level of the capillary blood. In metabolic acidosis, hyperventilation can occur very quickly because of the effect of H^+ ions on breathing. The P_aCO_2 typically decreases by 1.2 mmHg (0.16 kPa) for each mEq/L drop in HCO_3^- below the normal value of 24 mEq/L.

C. ACCEPTABLE ALVEOLAR VENTILATION WITH pH VARIATIONS

Metabolic alkalosis (P_aCO_2 30 to 50 mmHg (4.0 to 6.7 kPa) and pH > 7.50). In this situation lung function is acceptable. There is simply a net loss of acid with a relative excess of HCO_3^-. Metabolic alkalosis occurs in several instances. Critically ill patients are often mildly alkalotic. A loss of hydrochloric acid from the stomach is responsible for the metabolic alkalosis observed secondary to protracted vomiting and nasogastric suctioning. If these patients receive corticosteroid medication, this often accelerates the retention of sodium by the distal convoluted kidney tubules. This may manifest itself in an increased renal excretion of K^+ and H^+ ions sufficient to initiate alkalosis.

Another interesting example involves hypokalemic alkalosis, caused by chronic intravenous fluid therapy without adequate potassium ion $[K^+]$ replacement. The mechanism explaining hypokalemic alkalosis relates to the concept of electroneutrality. The normal intracellular $[K^+]$ is 130 to 140 mEq/L. Any depletion of $[K^+]$ in the extracellular fluid is replenished by a shift of K^+ from the intracellular to the extracellular fluid compartments. Electroneutrality in the cells is maintained by simultaneous movement of H^+ ions from the extracellular to intracellular compartments, but the extracellular fluid becomes alkalotic in the process.

Certain diuretic agents function very well to increase urine output, but also cause ion imbalances of a nature which initiate alkalosis. Many diuretics prevent Na^+ reabsorption from the kidney tubules into the bloodstream. In the proximal convoluted tubule normally 65% of the Na^+ ions are reabsorbed along with Cl^- ions, and an osmotic equivalent of water. Another 20% of the Na^+ ions are reabsorbed in exchange for H^+ and K^+ ions. Blockage of these proximal tubule reabsorption mechanisms keeps water from entering the circulation, thus promoting diuresis, but initiates a hypochloremia and hyponatremia. This is sensed by the adrenal cortex, which liberates aldosterone, and increases the amount of Na^+ ions reabsorbed at the distal convoluted tubule. Here H^+ ions are exchanged for Na^+ ions, thus an alkalosis can occur. But as the $[H^+]$ of these cells diminishes, K^+ ions are excreted instead, causing a secondary hypokalemia. If untreated, this in itself can be dangerous because of the importance of optimal Na^+/K^+ ratios in tension-generating muscle, especially the heart.

The treatment for most of these metabolic alkaloses is simply replacement of K^+, Cl^-, and water. The kidneys then attempt to bring the alkalotic blood pH to more normal levels.

Metabolic acidosis (P_aCO_2 30 to 50 mmHg (4.0 to 6.7 kPa) and pH < 7.50). Here, although the P_aCO_2 is acceptable, there is a well-defined acidosis. For reasons that would require additional information to interpret adequately, the ventilatory system has not responded to compensate for the metabolic acidosis.

D. VENTILATORY FAILURE WITH pH VARIATIONS

Partially compensated metabolic alkalosis ($P_aCO_2 > 50$ mmHg (6.7 kPa) and pH > 7.50). An increased P_aCO_2 often implies CO_2 accumulation from ventilatory failure. In this instance the unacceptably high pH indicates that the fundamental problem is a metabolic alkalosis to which the body is responding by decreasing ventilatory activity. However, the decreased ventilation here is inadequate to return the pH to acceptable limits. In asthmatic patients the P_aCO_2 may rise even above 100 mmHg.

Chronic ventilatory failure ($P_aCO_2 > 50$ mmHg (6.7 kPa) and pH 7.30 to 7.50). The pH maintenance within normal limits despite an elevated P_aCO_2 indicates that this is a manageable (chronic) situation where renal retention of HCO_3^- is assisting adequately with what is primarily a failure of the pulmonary system.

Acute ventilatory failure ($P_aCO_2 > 50$ mmHg (6.7 kPa) and pH < 7.30. The unacceptably low pH in the face of an elevated P_aCO_2 from failing ventilation indicates that this must be an acute situation, as yet uncompensated for by the kidney due to its short duration.

Examples of respiratory acidosis. The many examples of respiratory acidosis can be grouped generally under four categories. One category involves a depression of the activity of central nervous system respiratory control centers (see Chapter Eleven). Barbiturate anesthesia might do this. So could brain trauma, or increases in cerebrospinal fluid pressure.

A second category involves situations where the brain breathing centers are functioning properly, but the neurons or neuromuscular junctions that connect to the muscles of ventilation are affected. Quadriplegia, for example, above the level of third cervical vertebra causes impairment or loss of phrenic nerve function. The drugs curare and succinylcholine are specific neuromuscular blocking agents for skeletal muscles, including the diaphragm. Native Indians in the jungles of Panama have been known to use curare-tipped darts to spear animals for food, killing their prey by causing ventilatory muscle failure. Botulinum toxin acts similarly. Myasthenia gravis is a neuromuscular disease of possible viral cause, which also affects ventilatory muscle function.

Lung diseases form a very important third category. These include chronic obstructive pulmonary disease, pneumonia, pulmonary emphysema, asthma, and respiratory distress syndrome.

A final category involves a hodgepodge of situations not covered by the other three groupings. Although neuromuscular function may not be diseased, and although the lungs themselves are healthy, still the ventilatory mechanism cannot function adequately. Severe obesity is one example. A pneumothorax is another. Pleural effusion is a third.

ASSESSING OXYGENATION STATUS IN THE CONTEXT OF ACID-BASE REGULATION

Ventilation and oxygenation are very different entities. Whereas P_aCO_2 directly reflects the adequacy of alveolar ventilation, the oxygen content of blood indicates its oxygenation status. Adequate ventilation involves the provision of adequate oxygen into the arterial blood and removing sufficient carbon dioxide from the mixed venous blood to permit normal metabolic function. Adequate oxygenation involves the provision of sufficient oxygen from arterial blood into all the metabolizing cells of the body, thereby ensuring their normal function. There are three important variables to be considered in blood oxygen transport.

A. ARTERIAL PO$_2$

The P_aO_2 represents dissolved O_2 and is the primary determinant of the O_2 gradient that will exist between peripheral capillaries and each of the cells that will receive it. The larger this concentration gradient, the faster O_2 will be able to enter the tissue cells and ensure adequate tissue metabolism. If P_aO_2 is unacceptably low, then tissue hypoxia is almost certain. An acceptable P_aO_2 is > 80 mmHg (10.6 kPa) whereas the normal (mean) P_aO_2 is 97 mmHg (12.9 kPa). The reason for such a large discrepancy between normal values and the low end of the acceptable range is that, even a P_aO_2 of 80 mmHg (10.6 kPa) will permit 90% saturation of hemoglobin molecule with O_2.

When the P_aO_2 drops below 80 mmHg, the term *hypoxemia* is used to indicate this unacceptable blood oxygenation status. Whereas a P_aO_2 of < 80 mmHg is considered *mild hypoxemia*, a P_aO_2 of < 70 mmHg (9.3 kPa) is *moderate hypoxemia*, and a P_aO_2 of < 60 mmHg (8 kPa) is considered *severe hypoxemia*.

If supplemental O_2 is used to raise the P_aO_2, thereby attempting to correct hypoxemia, three additional descriptive terms are used to describe its effectiveness. If supplemental O_2 has raised the P_aO_2 between 80 and 100 mmHg, then the hypoxemia is *corrected*. If the P_aO_2 still has not reached acceptable limits, the hypoxemia is *uncorrected*. If the P_aO_2 is > 100 mmHg, the hypoxemia is *excessively corrected*.

Remember that, by definition, hypoxemia represents a P_aO_2 < 80 mmHg (10.6 kPa) when the subject is breathing room air. Hypoxemia does not guarantee tissue hypoxia, but certainly suggests the possibility. Hypoxemia coupled with acidemia virtually assures that tissue hypoxia exists. It would be inappropriate and possibly dangerous to discontinue oxygen therapy just to determine unequivocally that arterial hypoxemia existed. The use of supplemental oxygen suggests hypoxemia.

B. HEMOGLOBIN-OXYGEN AFFINITY

This topic was discussed thoroughly in Chapter Nine; however, a brief summary of important points concerning it and acid-base regulation are appropriate. The binding affinity of hemoglobin for O_2 is very strong, and unless three ligands are present in sizeable quantity, inadequate supplies of O_2 would be released to sustain life. Interestingly, all three of these ligands are products of metabolism, and acidic: CO_2, H^+ ions themselves, and 2,3-diphosphoglyceric acid. Thus, wherever the body requires increased O_2 delivery to tissues during states of elevated metabolism (fever, exercise, etc.), the increasing acidosis accompanying this rising metabolism allows greater hemoglobin deoxygenation.

The acidosis-induced change in position of the oxyhemoglobin dissociation curve that occurs when the percent saturation of hemoglobin is plotted against arterial PO_2—known as the Bohr shift to the right—allows quantitation of this O_2 release. Acidosis increases the P_{50} value of hemoglobin. These concepts were discussed in Chapter Nine.

As hemoglobin loses its O_2, its ability to bind CO_2 and H^+ increases. Reduced (or hydrogenated) hemoglobin thus serves as a very important buffer, allowing for the transport of sizable quantities of acid without lowering arterial pH.

C. BLOOD O_2 CONTENT

Oxygen content of the blood is determined by the sum of dissolved O_2 (P_aO_2) and bound O_2 (HbO_2). It is difficult to assess exactly which of the two is of greater importance from the standpoint of acid-base regulation, even though bound O_2

typically contributes 98.5% of the total blood O_2 transported. Hemoglobin is a very important buffer in addition to an O_2 reservoir. Yet, without the gradient of O_2 flow to tissues, set up by dissolved O_2, diffusion would not occur. As P_aO_2 decreases, O_2 leaves its hemoglobin reservoir and enters the dissolved state. The two forms of O_2 carriage are thus inseparably linked. Any decrease in blood levels of hemoglobin, brought about by problems such as chronic hemolysis, iron deficiency, or blood loss might lead to anemia. Thus, not only hypoxemia but also anemia will decrease blood O_2 content.

RELEVANT READING

Burke, M.D. Blood gas measurements, *Postgraduate Medicine* **64**(6): 163–167, 1978.

Davenport, H.W. *The ABC of Acid-Base Chemistry* (6th Ed.). Chicago: University of Chicago Press, 124 pp., 1980.

Dill, D.B. and Henderson, L.J. his transition from physical chemist to physiologist; his qualities as a man. *Physiologist* **20**(2):1–15, 1977.

Flenley, D.C. Blood gas and acid-base interpretation. *Respiratory Care* **27**:311–317, 1982.

Hasselbalch, K.A. Die Berechnung der Wasserstoffzahl des Blutes aus der freien und gebundenen Kohlensaure desselben, und die Sauerstoffbindung des Blutes als Funktion der Wasserstoffzahl. *Biochemische Zeitschrift* **78**:112–114, 1916.

Henderson, L.J. The theory of neutrality regulation in the animal organism. *American Journal of Physiology* **21**:427–448, 1908.

Hood, I., and Campbell, E.J.M. Is pk OK? *New England Journal of Medicine* **306**:864–865, 1982.

Kassirer, J.P., and Madias, N.E. Respiratory acid-base disorders. *Hospital Practice* **15**(12):57–71, 1980.

Meeroff, J.C., Penrock, B.E., and Llach, F. Rapid conversion of pH to [H+]. *Hospital Practice* **16**(1):71, 1981.

Milhorn, H.T. Understanding arterial blood gases. *American Family Physician* **21**(3):112–120, 1980.

Siggaard-Andersen, O. Blood acid-base alignment nomogram. *Scandinavian Journal of Clinical and Laboratory Investigation* **15**:211–217, 1963.

Shapiro, B. A., Harrison, R. A., and Walton, J.R. *Clinical Application of Blood Gases* Chicago: Year Book Medical Publishers, Inc., 3rd Ed., 316 pp., 1982.

Regulation of Breathing

Chapter Eleven

Chapter Eleven Outline

Central Nervous System Control

    A. Anatomical Aspects of Brainstem Ventilatory Control

    B. The Fundamental Stimulus for Breathing

Peripheral Arterial Control

    A. Anatomical and Operational Aspects

    B. Practical Considerations

        1. Anemia

        2. Hemorrhage

        3. Carbon Monoxide Poisoning

        4. Anesthesia

        5. Ascent to High Altitude

Other Influences on Breathing

    A. Cerebral Cortical Influences

    B. Valsalva-Related Influences

    C. Nasal Reflexes and Sneezing

    D. Laryngeal-Tracheal Reflexes and Coughing

    E. Vomiting Reflex and its Ventilatory Modification

    F. Diaphragm Spasm and Hiccuping

    G. Lung Epithelial Irritant Receptors

    H. Alveolar Nociceptive Reflexes

    I. Pulmonary Stretch Receptors and Hering-Breuer Reflex

    J. Other Ventilatory Pattern Alterations

    K. Ventilation During Exercise

Breathing, just as the beating of the heart, is an ongoing process which seems to regulate itself to meet body needs. Only a moment of thought, however, will reveal that many factors can alter the breathing pattern, including a major component from the cerebral cortex. There is a great variety, both voluntary and involuntary, of breathing patterns. Irritants can cause coughing or sneezing or vomiting, which affect the respiratory muscles and alter the breathing patterns remarkably. A rise in body temperature increases frequency and decreases tidal volume.

There is the obvious conclusion that a fundamental driving nervous mechanism must set the basic pattern, but that a sizable number of other distinct control mechanisms all interconnect with this system. Despite a hundred years of research, there are still many major questions yet remaining, which will explain the role of blood chemicals, such as CO_2 and H^+ ions, the role of nervous activity arising from the periphery and impacting on the central drive mechanism, the role of irritants in the respiratory tract on the total picture of breathing, and the altered breathing patterns brought about by specific diseases. This Chapter provides an introductory survey of some of these areas of interest.

CENTRAL NERVOUS SYSTEM CONTROL

A. ANATOMICAL ASPECTS OF BRAINSTEM VENTILATORY CONTROL

The typical breathing pattern of resting humans has two phases: inspiration, which requires about one second, and then, when inspiration is finished, more quickly than it began it ceases, with a period of expiratory silence more variant in duration, lasting as long as 3 to 4 times the inspiratory phase.

Even though many physiological characteristics may be altered by factors such as fever, hypoxia, and acidosis, the same *basic rhythm* or pattern is maintained. Thus, the basic rhythm is not necessarily determined by fluctuations in core temperature, or blood gas concentrations, or body pH. Rather, it is modified by such changes.

Ventilatory patterns of dogs and cats, who have had a transection which severs connections from either the cerebral cortex or the cerebellum to the rest of their brain, are essentially unchanged from the normal pattern. This implies that the basic rhythm must be generated within the remainder of the brain and spinal cord, with areas such as the cerebral cortex and cerebellum having modifying or modulating influences. A transection to sever connections between the spinal cord and the medulla oblongata of the brainstem eliminates the basic ventilatory rhythm, suggesting rather strongly that the brainstem must be the source of the neural respiratory drive. Years of research have been directed toward identifying where these neurons might be, and how they interact. One plausible hypothesis is that 1) some trigger occurs that initially activates the inspiratory neurons, 2) there are inspiratory neurons, which when stimulated, result in phrenic nerve activation, 3) expiratory neurons in some way inhibit the inspiratory neurons and thus generate the actual rhythm, and 4) as inspiration occurs, there is communication to the expiratory neurons to keep them "informed" of their impending need to become more active. It has been a difficult endeavor to match facts with hypothesis, and to match signals obtained by neurophysiologial experiments with neuroanatomical pathways.

Figure 11-1 provides one version of a useful scheme for comprehending in general terms the controlling mechanisms in breathing. The automaticity of breathing rhythm resides in the medulla oblongata. Modifying influences on this rhythm come voluntarily from the cerebral cortex, and involuntarily from input via the pons (a region above the medulla that forms a connecting bridge between cerebellum and brainstem) and spinal cord. The primary sensor that initiates inspiration is chemical, and is described in greater detail in the following section. A sizable array of other factors—stretch receptors in the lung and pleura, proprioreceptors in the joints, peripheral baroreceptors, and more—all affect the eventual strength of the breathing stimulus.

Beyond this general picture, it is difficult to be precise in defining specific neural cell types and pathways that explain how breathing is controlled. In part this is because the picture is far from clearly understood. Also, experimental data from non-human species often do not apply specifically to the differing neuroanatomical and neurophysiological picture found in the human brain.

Three specific regions in the brainstem have been identified. A dorsal respiratory group of neurons is positioned bilaterally in the medulla, with activities geared preferentially toward initiation of inspiration. A ventral respiratory group of neurons is located in the ventrolateral brainstem as a long continuous bilateral column of cells. Its more rostral portion has neurons which preferentially influence inspiration. The more caudal portion has primarily neurons which influence expiration. Finally, above both groups, in the dorsolateral rostral pons, lies a region called the pneumotaxic center, long known for its relationship to breathing. Lesions there produce apneusis—prolonged inspirations, as long as 4 minutes.

The exact details of how these various neuron groups interact or modify the basic inspiratory rhythm are still being sought. One concept of neuronal function, that of reciprocal inhibition, is probably involved. That is, neuron A inhibits neuron B, and neuron B inhibits neuron A. But that is insufficient. Neuron A and/or neuron B must be affected by other neurons. Another concept, that of recurrent excitation and inhibition—where a particular neuronal output increases or decreases the activity of other neurons—is also likely involved.

THE FUNDAMENTAL STIMULUS FOR BREATHING

The fundamental trigger for generation of inspiration is accumulation of CO_2 or acid in the brain. The initial experimental evidence for this finding arose with

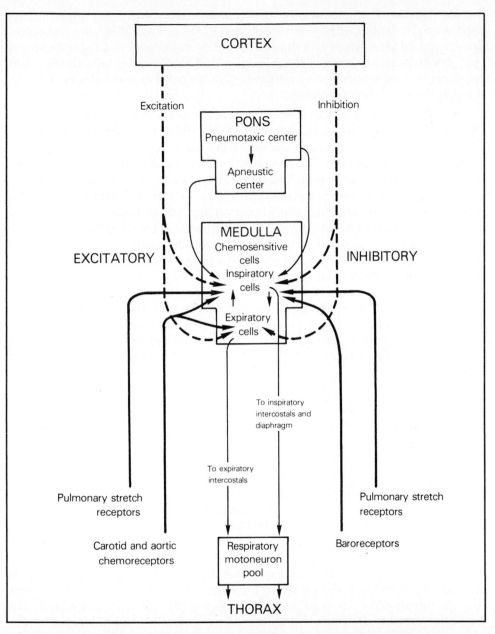

Figure 11-1. Diagram of central and peripheral aspects of control of breathing. What at first appears a rather simple process, namely the maintenance of a rhythmic breathing pattern, is an extremely complicated process, involving aspects of blood chemistry, neuromuscular coordination, and moment-to-moment changes characteristic of life itself. (Reprinted with permission from *Neurogenic factors in control of respiration*, by C.J. Lambertsen, Ch. 38, in Medical Physiology (V.B. Mountcastle, ed.), p. 704, 12th Ed., C.V. Mosby Co., St. Louis, 1968).

the observation that perfusion of the cerebral brain ventricles with simulated cerebrospinal fluid (CSF) containing a high CO_2 or elevated H^+ ion concentration increased breathing. Perfusion with fluid containing a low CO_2 or decreased H^+ concentration depressed it. This suggested that certain cells in the brain, sensitive to the chemical composition of CSF, respond to maintain its chemical stability by regulating breathing.

How do arterial blood PCO_2 and H^+ ions, or brain PCO_2 or H^+, affect CSF PCO_2 and H^+ ions? Carbon dioxide, being freely diffusible, moves rapidly across the blood-brain and blood-cerebrospinal fluid barriers, whereas H^+ and HCO_3^- ions do not. Thus, the PCO_2 of cerebrospinal fluid and internal jugular venous blood are approximately equal. Thus, inhalation of CO_2 leads immediately to an increase in P_aCO_2 of cerebrospinal fluid (CSF). This fluid differs from blood in many ways, particularly in its lacking a protein buffer system such as hemoglobin. There is also no carbonic anhydrase present. Thus, when CO_2 enters CSF, it slowly becomes hydrated to form H_2CO_3, which in turn dissociates into H^+ and HCO_3^- ions. Neurons in the wall of the fourth ventricle, which are bathed with CSF and sensitive to increased levels of H^+ ions, respond to this stimulus by increasing action potential traffic to the medullary inspiratory area. These stimuli sum together with all the other incoming impulses to this region. The total motor response of this inspiratory area is designed to bring about an appropriate inspiratory response that ultimately will maintain the partial pressure of CO_2 in the cerebrospinal fluid constant, and with it, a constant CSF pH.

Chronic obstructive pulmonary disease causes a prolonged increase in P_aCO_2, and thus a chronic increase in the $P_{CSF}CO_2$. This should produce a chronically elevated $[H^+]$ and $[HCO_3^-]$ in CSF, and with it a chronically increased breathing stimulus. With time, however, the sensitivity of the chemosensitive cells to these elevated H^+ levels decreases, decreasing the magnitude of the breathing stimulus, and making it mandatory for other mechnisms to stimulate breathing to assist. These peripheral mechanisms will be discussed in the following section.

Hyperventilation will result in a lowered P_aCO_2, and an individual can breathhold for a longer period of time than normal. The central driving system lowers its activity level. Since CO_2 is the primary driving stimulus for breathing, the rate decreases. The relative ineffectiveness of hypoxia as a central stimulus when compared to hypercapnia is unfortunately dramatized when, as a stunt or because of a challenge from friends, a swimmer hyperventilates prior to attempting an underwater swim, for example, to transverse the length of a pool. Hyperventilation lowers CO_2 but does little to raise oxygen levels in the blood. The swimmer extracts O_2 from the blood, and eventually cerebral hypoxia may induce unconsciousness prior to CO_2 accumulation in sufficient quantity to force the swimmer to surface. When this occurs, voluntary breathing-holding ceases, and water may enter the lungs if reflexive laryngospasm does not ensue first.

While the effectiveness of carbon dioxide as a ventilatory stimulus to drive the central oscillatory breathing mechanism cannot be denied, knowledge is still lacking that explains how the rhythmic oscillatory breathing pattern occurs. It probably is neural rather than chemical. It is at least plausible to envision neural monitoring of neural signals with inhibition increasing as excitation increases. It is less simple to imagine breath-by-breath monitoring, at the medullary level, of gas-exchange dynamics occurring at the alveolocapillary membrane level, displaced not only in distance but also in time. Nevertheless, its effectiveness is so extraordinary that in a healthy individual the P_aCO_2 does not vary much more than about 3 mmHg (0.4 kPa) over the course of a day.

PERIPHERAL ARTERIAL CONTROL

A. ANATOMICAL AND OPERATIONAL ASPECTS

In addition to the central system for regulation of ventilation, there is an important peripheral system involving specialized chemosensitive cells. These are in the aortic bodies, attached to the arch of the aorta, and in the carotid bodies, small pinkish nodules located at the bifurcation of each common carotid artery into the external and internal carotids.

Anatomists have been aware of the carotid bodies since 1743. It wasn't until 1928, however, that deCastro identified their probable chemoreceptive function. In 1929 the Belgian father-son scientific team of Corneille and J.F. Heymans reported that blood low in O_2 or high in CO_2, when present in the left ventricle and first part of the aorta, would stimulate increased breathing provided that the vagus nerves were intact. Heymans later described similar chemosensitive zones in the carotid arteries; these became known as carotid bodies. The identification of these structures and delineation of their function, were such important milestones in the development of physiology that the Nobel Prize in medicine and physiology was conferred upon Heymans in 1938 for his work.

Afferent neurons from both the carotid sinus and carotid body ascend as part of the carotid nerve to join the glossopharyngeal nerve (Figures 11-2, 11-3). Cell bodies for these neurons are located in the petrosal ganglion, which contains all the cell bodies of neurons comprising the ninth cranial nerve. The aortic bodies contain chemoreceptors that function separately from the aortic arch baroreceptors, which are in the wall of the ascending arch of the aorta. Most of the aortic chemoreceptors lie between the arch of the aorta and the pulmonary artery or on the dorsal aspect of the pulmonary artery. The afferent nerve fibers from the aortic bodies enter the vagal nerve pathways usually along with the recurrent laryngeal nerves. Their cell bodies are in the nodose ganglia of the vagus nerves.

It seems probable that the carotid and aortic bodies in man represent the survival of structures of great importance in the control of ventilation in water breathing forms. It is logical that O_2-consuming animals living in water would desire sensitive detecting mechanisms for hypoxic (low PO_2) or hypercapnic (high PCO_2) fluid environments. The logical site for such organs would be at the

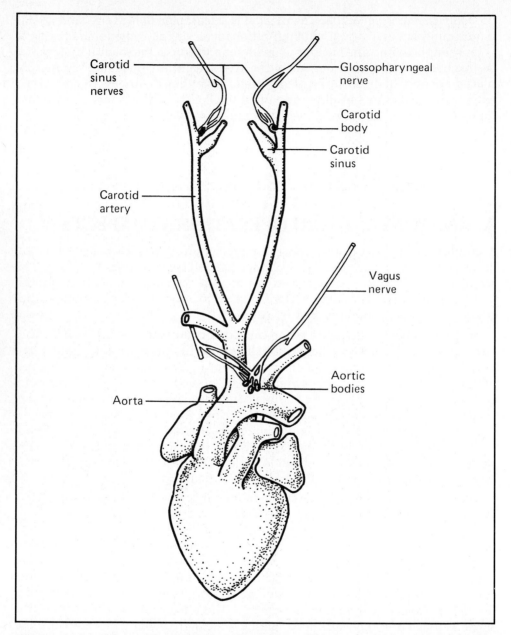

Figure 11-2. The aortic and carotid bodies with their connecting innervations to nearby cranial nerves (vagus for aortic bodies, glosso-pharyngeal for carotid bodies).

place where salt water or fresh water contacts the bloodstream. Embryologically, the carotid body is associated with the third bronchial arch, the aortic body with the fourth. These are the ontogenetic equivalents to the phylogenetic third and fourth gill arches of fishes. Just as the gill movements of fishes are more sensitive to decreased PO_2 than to increased PCO_2 in the surrounding water, so then it might be expected that the chemoreceptors in man would be preferentially hypoxia-sensitive rather than hypercapnia-sensitive. In man the aortic body is much less sensitive than the carotid body as a chemoreceptor; if it could be removed, its function is scarcely missed.

The mechanism by which hypoxia or hypercapnia is translated into afferent nerve impulses is presently being elucidated. Apparently, there are glomus cells, which in fact are neurons, located within the carotid body. They produce the neurotransmitter dopamine, which here is inhibitory, and they synapse with carotid nerve fibers. Thus, there is a kind of reciprocal synapse. The carotid sinus nerve cells tend to activate glomus cells through release of acetylcholine, and these glomus cells in turn inhibit the carotid sinus nerve cells through the action of dopamine.

The key to understanding chemoreceptor function is to understand how hypoxia and hypercapnia alter this relatively steady-state interneuronal equilibrium. It seems best to characterize the stimulus as a decrease in O_2 supply below the needs of these highly metabolic cells (or an increase in CO_2 surrounding them). Thus, a normal blood flow but a low P_aO_2 would be an effective stimulus. Also would be a decreased blood flow but a normal P_aO_2.

These arterial chemoreceptors have extraordinarily high metabolic rates, requiring enormous blood flow on a ml/gm tissue basis. This blood flow is achieved by having tortuous anastomosing sinusoids on the arterial side of each chemoreceptor, where perfusing pressure is high. The flow is about 20 ml/gm tissue/min (compared to approximately 1.4 ml/gm heart tissue/min or 1.7 ml/gm brain tissue/min).

There is, of course, tonic activity in these chemoreceptors, since they are living cells. Their noticeable effects on ventilation, which would be superimposed on the central nervous system oscillation, begin to appear when the equivalent of mixed venous blood—in terms of PO_2 and PCO_2—begins to perfuse them. A P_aO_2 of about 70 mmHg (9.3 kPa), or a P_aCO_2 exceeding 44 mmHg (5.9 kPa) provides a greater-than-normal stimulus to the afferent nerves involved, with a pronounced increase in breathing rate and depth.

These activational constraints imply that in healthy people, whether at rest or during exercise, at sea level, and even at altitudes as high as 8,000 or 9,000 feet (2,438 to 2,743 m) chemoreceptors would have little more than tonic baseline activity. However, in patients with respiratory disease, P_aO_2 values less than 70 mmHg (9.3 kPa) can be encountered frequently. In such patients the carotid bodies form a major driving force for breathing. Often, in such patients, their chronic acidosis eventually results in normalization of the cerebrospinal fluid pH via bicarbonate adjustment, in turn reducing the vigor of the central chemoreceptor driving mechanism. Bilateral carotid body resection would not be advisable in such patients because a sizeable portion of their breathing-control system would be lost.

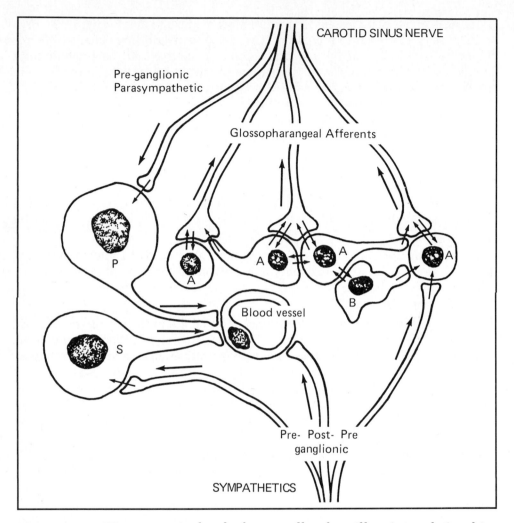

Figure 11-3. Diagrammatic sketch of nerve cell and capillary interrelationships in the rat carotid body. A and B are two different types of carotid body (or glomus) cells. P and S represent parasympathetic and sympathetic ganglion cells whose action regulated blood flow through local capillaries. Afferent neurons, which are chemosensitive, constitute the carotid sinus nerve, which eventually merges with the glossopharyngeal nerve sending information to the medulla oblongata. In some areas there are synapses with reciprocal activity (inhibition/excitation)—see the double arrows. (Reprinted with permission from McDonald DM, and Mitchell, R.A., *Journal of Neurocytology* 4:177–230, 1975).

B. PRACTICAL CONSIDERATIONS

The arterial chemoreceptors act as part of a dual sensing system capable jointly of detecting changes both in the environment of the central neurons and in the arterial blood that has just been exposed to the pulmonary gas exchange process. Either component of this sensing system is capable of driving ventilation when the other component is no longer capable of independent function. The peripheral sensing mechnism is able to respond to changes in more than one chemical factor. The ultimate purpose of both systems is to maintain the acid-base environment most suitable for central function and the oxygenation of the arterial blood supply to the body tissues. Several examples of departures from normal health at a sea level environment can illustrate how the systems interact.

1. *Anemia*

Patients with severe anemia do not experience ventilatory stimulation at rest, even though their blood hemoglobin levels may be very low. If their lung function, P_AO_2, P_aO_2, and peripheral chemoreceptor blood flow are all normal, the CO_2 of blood bathing the peripheral chemoreceptor cells will not drop, and its PCO_2 will not rise. Neither mechanism for increasing respiration will be activated. The enormous needs of the peripheral chemoreceptors regarding O_2 are still met.

2. *Hemorrhage*

A marked decrease in blood flow can cause hypoxia in the peripheral chemoreceptor cells even though P_aO_2 and O_2 content are normal. Blood flow may be reduced either because the pressure in the systemic arteries is low, as a result of severe hemorrhage, or because the arterioles supplying the chemoreceptors have constricted even though arterial blood pressure is reasonably high. A decrease in blood flow to one-fourth normal does not lower tissue PO_2 nearly as much as hypoxemia with normal blood flow. The carotid body, however, appears to suffer to about the same extent. This unexpected activity is likely caused by an accumulation—because of decreased flow—of metabolically produced CO_2 which, via H^+ ions, vigorously stimulates these peripheral chemoreceptor cells.

3. *Carbon Monoxide Poisoning*

Patients with carbon monoxide (CO) poisoning do not exhibit increased breathing. Because of a 200 to 250 fold greater affinity of CO than O_2 for hemoglobin, this means than only ½00 to ½50 as much CO as O_2 is required in inspired air for the two gases to compete on even terms for hemoglobin. Thus, 0.02% CO added to the inspired air would reduce the inspired oxygen from 20.93% to 20.91%, yet still would result in 50% of the hemoglobin binding sites for O_2 being occupied by CO. The P_IO_2 decreases from 159.0 mmHg to 158.5 mmHg. P_ICO_2 is unaffected. Peripheral chemoreceptors are not stimulated because P_aO_2 is still high. Yet, there is a dramatic reduction in arterial O_2 content. The resulting cerebral hypoxemia results in cerebral tissue hypoxia sufficient to cause unconsciousness. This is a special situation where an infinitesimal reduction in P_aO_2 can still induce a marked decrease in arterial O_2 content.

4. *Anesthesia*

During anesthesia the central respiratory centers can become hypoxic, and depressed in their sensitivity of response. The peripheral chemoreceptors, by contrast, increase their response during hypoxic states, and can overcome the depressant effect on ventilation by additional peripheral activation, via their carotid and glossopharyngeal nerve connections, to the brain respiratory centers.

5. *Ascent to High Altitude*

When one quickly travels to an altitude sufficient to lower the P_aO_2 of blood perfusing the arterial chemoreceptors to about 70 mmHg (9.3 kPa), their stimulation elicits an increased ventilation. This is a hyperventilation and not a hyperpnea, because general body metabolism may have increased only slightly. The hyperventilation decreases P_ACO_2, P_aCO_2, and $P_{CSF}CO_2$. The arterial blood pH and cerebrospinal fluid pH both rise slightly, and since the central chemoreceptors are primarily H^+ receptors, they decrease somewhat their excitation of the medullary respiratory center, lowering the respiratory rate toward normal. At such altitudes of 10,000 feet (3,280 meters) or greater, the peripheral chemoreceptors have a greater influence on control of breathing.

Upon return to sea level following several weeks of altitude residence, mild hypoventilation will occur, for the first few days. The hypoxemic peripheral chemoreceptor drive has been removed and the central chemoreceptor mechanism is not quite as active as previously. During this readaptive period many people feel noticeably sluggish. Carbon dioxide accumulation occurs, and the rapid movement of this into the cerebrospinal fluid soon causes a marked decrease in its $[H^+]$. The central chemoreceptors are now stimulated to an extent greater than that normally seen at sea level, and respiration increases. Gradual active transport of bicarbonate into the cerebrospinal fluid restores the fluid pH back to its usual value of about 7.32, and normal respiration resumes.

Three large cities in the United States are at altitudes high enough to be at the threshold of response to altitude hypoxia: Albuquerque, Colorado Springs, and Denver. A typical P_B in those cities might be 600 mm Hg (80 kPa), with a P_aO_2 of about 77 mmHg (10 kPa), a P_aCO_2 of about 37 mm Hg (4.9 kPa), and a slightly increased erythrocyte concentration.

OTHER INFLUENCES ON BREATHING

While the central chemoreceptor drive in normal man represents the ongoing means for permitting rhythmic ventilation to occur, there are several significant influences that can modify this rhythm. Some are central, some peripheral, and still others arise from alterations in body activity patterns, a common example being exercise.

A. *Cerebral Cortical Influences*

The normal ventilatory rhythm can be voluntarily accelerated or slowed. Thus, one presumes that both cortical excitatory and inhibitory neural input to the brainstem respiratory centers can occur. The simplest arrangement would be for these inputs to directly influence the inspiratory and expiratory cells of the medulla.

One can voluntarily hyperventilate sufficiently to raise the arterial blood pH by 0.2 unit, and a P_aCO_2 reduction from 45 mmHg (6.0 kPa) to 25 mmHg (3.3 kPa) is not unreasonable. By reviewing the graphical relationship between blood PCO_2, HCO_3^- and pH in Chapter Ten this can be more easily appreciated.

B. Valsalva-Related Influences

When performing such voluntary acts as laughing, speaking, singing, musical horn blowing, etc., the normal breathing pattern is also disrupted, with more or less prolonged periods of hypoventilation. The usual hypercapnic stimulus to breathe prevails, with breathing eventually resuming, but because these are voluntary acts, the cerebral cortex is actively involved. Most of these activities all involve as well a movement pattern commonly called the Valsalva maneuver, named after the 17th century Italian anatomist, Antonio Valsalva who first described it.

When the glottis is voluntarily closed, and the abdominal and thoracic expiratory muscles activated, intra-thoracic and intra-abdominal pressures will rise, and ventilation ceases. This maneuver is used during defecation and childbirth. There is very little stress on the alveoli or the air ducts because the pressure is being generated by the thoracic and abdominal muscles. But the high intrathoracic pressure decreases or stops venous return to the heart. Systemic blood pressure initially rises because of the increased intrathoracic pressure, but then falls as the cardiac output decreases because of a decrease in venous return. While the intra-thoracic and intra-abdominal arteries are not stressed during this maneuver, the arteries of the anus, leg, head, and superficial trunk are stressed because the intra-arterial pressure rises without any increase in external supporting pressure. The rise in intrathoracic and intra-abdominal pressures causes a rise in cerebrospinal fluid pressure due to transmission of the pressure change through the intervertebral foramina. This rise in cerebrospinal fluid pressure can place stress on the intracranial vessels.

C. Nasal Reflexes and Sneezing

Sneezing is a reflex response elicited by irritation of the mucous membrane of the nasal mucosa. Water, noxious gases, and cigarette smoke are all effective stimuli. Impulses ascend into the brain via the trigeminal and facial nerves and make synaptic connections with the appropriate tracts leading out of the brain to the ventilatory muscles. There is an initial inspiration and then an explosive expiration. It is presumed that the medullary expiratory neurons are stimulated because the accessory ventilatory muscles, activated during high-flow breathing, are involved.

D. Laryngeal-Tracheal Reflexes and Coughing

When specific chemical or physical irritants pass below the larynx and into the trachea, a cough can be engendered. This is similar to the Valsalva maneuver—a high intrathoracic pressure is developed against a closed glottis. The

glottis is then opened abruptly, creating a large pressure gradient between alveolar pressure and upper tracheal pressure (atmospheric); this results in a very
rapid flow rate. During the explosive expiration there is a narrowing of the
trachea due to the high intrathoracic pressure. This inverts the non-cartilaginous
portion of the trachea such that the cross-sectional area is decreased by 85%. The
high linear velocity can reach 500 miles per hour (233 m/sec) and is particularly
well suited for the purpose of dislodging or expelling foreign material. It is
initiated in the mucosal receptors of the airways, which are innervated by the
vagus nerves. The most sensitive cough-producing areas are the larynx and
tracheal bifurcation into primary bronchi. Local anesthetic agents can paralyze
these receptors, but abolition of the cough reflex carries with it a substantial risk
of clogging the airways, with the typical sequelae of ventilatory disturbance and
initiation of infection.

E. Vomiting Reflex and its Ventilatory Modification

Vomiting is a complex reflex act. It is usually preceded by a feeling of sickness
or nausea and an active secretion of saliva. The saliva, mixed with air, accumulates to a considerable extent at the lower end of the esophagus and causes some
distention. A forced inspiration is made while the glottis remains open so that air
enters the lungs. Later, the glottis opening moves to redirect inspired air into the
esophagus. This adds to the distention already caused by the accumulated saliva.
The breath is held and the diaphragm depressed, with consequent straightening
of the esophagus. The abdominal muscles generate tension and compress the
stomach against the diaphragm; simultaneously the cardiac sphincter relaxes.
The head is held forward and the stomach contents are ejected through the
previously distended esophagus. Stomach compression by the shortening abdominal muscles supplies the force needed to eject the stomach contents. The
act of vomiting is controlled by a center located in the medulla known as the area
postrema, near the tractus solitarius, and the different fibers to this center may
come from many different regions of the body. Some arise from the sensory nerve
endings of the fauces (the narrow passage from the mouth to the pharynx situated
between the soft palate and the base of the tongue and bounded laterally by two
curved folds enclosing the tonsil on each side) and the pharynx. Other afferent
impulses come from the mucosa of the stomach and duodenum; these are excited
by most emetic agents. Certain emetics, such as apomorphine, are directly active
on the medullary vomiting center and can be given parenterally. Physical stimulation of the labyrinths of the ear sufficient to stimulate the vestibular pathways,
may also induce vomiting as a result of the connections of this nervous pathway
with these brain centers.

F. Diaphragm Spasm and Hiccuping

Hiccuping is an intermittent spasm of the diaphragm often accompanied by
similar tension generation in the accessory muscles of inspiration. It can occur in
a variety of disease situations but occurs in healthy individuals for no apparent
reason, or after specific incidents such as laughter. Its exact mechanism of origin
remains obscure. Both central and peripheral explanations have been pro-

posed—excitation of the phrenic nerve, the motor cortex, etc. One method for inhibiting hiccuping involves repeated swallowing. The mechanism acts directly on the medullary respiratory center to inhibit ventilation in that particular phase of the cycle. Since swallowing itself is a reflex act and does not occur unless there is a stimulus in the form of fluid or a bolus of food affecting the receptors in the back of the mouth, one common technique is to swallow very small portions of water continuously with no breath in between for about 20 to 30 seconds, beginning near the time of the next expected hiccuping episode.

G. Lung Epithelial Irritant Receptors

Reflex bronchoconstriction and hyperventilation can occur when smoke, dust, and other chemical irritants contact receptors extending from the trachea to the respiratory bronchioles. Coughing is not induced by activation of these specific irritant receptors. The receptor endings can actually penetrate the surface epithelium. The activating stimuli can also include pressure, such as by passage of an endobronchial catheter, and distortion of the wall of the airway by such diverse causes as pneumothorax, pulmonary congestion, and atelectasis. The vagus nerves mediate the observed reflex response.

H. Alveolar Nociceptive Reflexes

In the alveolar walls, near pulmonary capillaries, receptor endings are located, these are terminal endings of afferent vagal neurons. They sometimes are called J-receptors (for juxta-pulmonary capillary receptors), and probably function most effectively in relation to pathological alterations in the alveolar wall and pulmonary circulation rather than in healthy man. The reflex causes temporary apnea, and possibly bronchoconstriction.

I. Pulmonary Stretch Receptors and the Hering-Breuer Reflex

A dramatic change in ventilation occurs in anesthetized dogs and rabbits when both vagus nerves are cut in the neck. Tidal volume abruptly becomes maximal and the frequency of breathing slows. The animal acts as if it were inspiring and expiring its vital capacity with each breath. Hering and Breuer, who performed these early experiments, noted that maintained distention of the lungs of anesthetized animals decreased the frequency of an inspiratory effort. They showed this effect to be a reflex mediated in part by the vagus nerves. The obvious conclusion is that some sensory information must normally travel along the vagus nerves, which, by its central action, prevents maximal inflation. Presumably, the neural end result is a stopping of inspiration at a smaller volume, permitting expiration to occur earlier.

The probable role of these so-called Hering-Breuer or vagal stretch reflexes is to regulate the work of the ventilatory muscles in such a way that the greatest alveolar ventilation occurs for the least muscular effort. The impulses traveling in the vagal fibers are indeed inhibitory, because inflation of the lung leads to an increase in the frequency of electrical impulses in these afferent fibers. Simultaneously there is a decrease or cessation of the electrical activity of inspiratory muscles such as the two hemidiaphragms.

The receptors are in the airway smooth muscle. When activated, there is not only the inspiratory inhibition just described but also a relaxation of tracheo-bronchial smooth muscle. Unless the lung inflation is large in man, however, the inspiratory inhibition is not manifested as much as the tracheobronchial airway expansion. This may be a matter of timing, however, with the intrinsic medullary activity already terminating inspiration just as the pulmonary stretch reflex activity is becoming measurable.

One can demonstrate by breath-holding that the inflation reflex is able to inhibit central respiratory activity. The breath can be held longer, and to a higher level of P_ACO_2, if the lungs are inflated than if they are deflated.

J. Other Ventilatory Pattern Alterations

Sighing is a slow deep inspiration followed by a slow deep expiration. The result is a temporary increase in P_aO_2, decrease in P_aCO_2 and increased venous return to the heart. It serves to open collapsed alveoli and temporarily overcome bronchiolar constriction. Hence it is a valuable mechanism for periodically "cleaning" the lung, providing fresh air to hypoventilated alveoli, and rejuvenating the surfactant layer. Yawning is about as little understood as sighing. The cardiopulmonary results are same, but yawning appears to occur principally during states of decreased awareness caused by physical exhaustion or approaching sleep periods.

Panting is a tachypnea performed by animals attempting to maintain their central, or core, temperature. This rapid shallow breathing moves fresh air into and out of the anatomic dead space far more frequently than does normal breathing. It is a mechanism used to eliminate heat by animals who do not have sweating mechanisms. Man does not utilize this mechanism. When the core temperature is raised, nerve cells in the hypothalamus send stimulatory information to the respiratory centers and the tachypneic response results. Man solves this problem by cutaneous vasodilation and sweating. An animal in tachypnea will never be hyperventilating because there is less alveolar ventilation than in hyperpnea. There is adequate ventilation, however.

Cheyne-Stokes breathing is a regular waxing and waning of tidal volume and ventilatory frequency. Is is usually observed with cerebrovascular disease and heart failure, and its explanation is presently being debated. Either there is a neurologic abnormality—an excessively depressed or excitable respiratory center—or a cardiovascular abnormality—a prolonged circulation time. Since patients with Cheyne-Stokes respiration often have both types of ailment, it is difficult to ascertain the exact cause. The pattern is named after the two physicians who initially reported the pattern: John Cheyne, a Scotsman, and William Stokes, an Irishman.

K. Ventilation During Exercise

The increase in ventilation with an increase in endurance-type exercise is known essentially to all who have exercised. The metabolic aspects of exercise, as they relate to stimulation of breathing will be discussed in Chapter Twelve. This increased rate and depth is a hyperpnea, not a hyperventilation. It is very difficult to explain this hyperpnea, since alveolar ventilation matches metabolic needs so nicely that P_aCO_2 and P_ACO_2 values are unchanged, except at extremely high work loads. There are probably many contributing factors, each somewhat small in itself, but nevertheless significant. One involves proprioceptors in the joints and muscles of the limbs. Another involves a rise in core temperature as exercise progresses. A third includes the neurogenic stimuli occurring from anticipation of exercise, and excitement about performing the exercise. At levels of exercise that result in entry of lactate into the blood, the gradually decreasing blood pH provides an increased stimulus to the medullary respiratory centers. Although not yet investigated very well in man, there may be subtle augmentation of breathing on a breath-to-breath basis, regulated by arterial chemoreceptors as they are bathed by blood emerging from the lungs.

RELEVANT READING

Berger, AJ, Mitchell RA, and Severinghaus JW.: Regulation of Respiration. *New England Journal of Medicine*, **297**:92–97, 138–143, 194–201, 1977.

Bradley GW: Control of breathing pattern. *International Review of Physiology*, Vol. 14 (J.G. Widdicombe, ed.), University Park Press, Baltimore, 185–217, 1974.

Cherniak NS, and Longobardo GS.: Cheyne-Stokes Breathing. *New England Journal of Medicine*, **288**:952–957, 1973

Cohen MI.: Central determinants of respiratory rhythm. *Annual Review of Physiology*, **43**:91–104, 1981.

Feldman JL.: Interactions between brainstem respiratory neurons. *Federation Proceedings*, 40:2384–2388, 1981.

Kalia MP.: Anatomical organization of central respiratory neurons. *Annual Review of Physiology*, **43**:105–120, 1981.

Long SE, and Duffin J: The medullary respiratory neurons: A review. *Canadian Journal of Physiology and Pharmacology*, **62**:161–182, 1984.

Lugliani R, Whipp BJ, Seard C, and Wasserman K.: Effect of bilateral carotid-body resection on ventilatory control at rest and during exercise in man. *New England Journal of Medicine*, **285**:1105–1111, 1971.

Merrill EG.: Where are the real respiratory neurons? *Federation Proceedings*, **40**:2389–2394, 1974.

Pick J.: The discovery of the carotid body. *Journal of the History of Medicine*, **14**:61–73, 1959.

Richter DW, Ballantyne D, and Remmers JH: How is the respiratory rhythm generated? A model. *News in Physiological Sciences*, **1**:109–112, 1986.

Schmidt CF, and Comroe JH, Jr.: Functions of the carotid and aortic bodies. *Physiological Reviews,* **20:**115–157, 1940.

Torrance RW.: Arterial chemoreceptors. *International Review of Physiology,* Vol. 2 (J.G. Widdicombe, ed.), University Park Press, Baltimore, 247–271, 1974.

Widdicombe JG.: Reflex control of breathing. *International Review of Physiology,* Vol. 2 (J.G. Widdicombe, ed.), University Park Press, 273–301, 1974.

Exercise: A Ventilatory and Metabolic Challenge

Chapter Twelve

Chapter Twelve Outline

Exercise and the performance of vigorous work are stresses on the cardiovascular, pulmonary and musculoskeletal systems, which ordinarily are idling in the resting state. Metabolic energy-producing systems accelerate their activities in a responsive harmony with the intensity of the exercise or workload. Increasing physical work presents a challenge to the body's abilities to transport O_2 to working tissues, clear CO_2 from these tissues, preserve an optimum acid-base status, and ensure adequate energy supplies. The cardiovascular and pulmonary systems both play an integral role in allowing this accelerated activity to continue. By understanding these roles, it should be possible to identify the mechanisms for improving capacities to perform increased work or exercise. For laborers this can mean greater productivity. For an elite athlete, it could mean a world record or an Olympic medal. For all of us interested in living a vigorously healthy life, it can form the groundwork for a proper exercise program.

The past decade has witnessed an unprecedented increase in desire for greater physical fitness. The thought of completing a marathon run (26.2 miles; 42.195 km) was in the minds of a precious few in 1970. Presently, at least 600 such marathons, some having as many as 20 thousand runners, with 90% or more actually finishing the run, occur annually around the world. Along with lesser-intensity footraces, triathloning, hiking, cycling, walking, tennis, cross-country skiing, and other activities, millions of people are striving for improved health through a vigorously active lifestyle.

Physical fitness assessment and long-term physiological monitoring of these healthy people, as well as prescription of exercise to allow sensible further development of fitness, has given rise to a host of new job descriptions in the health care field. Respiratory therapists, physiologists, and cardiopulmonary technicians in particular are interacting extensively with physicians in this expanding new area. Understanding the cardiovascular and respiratory effects of exercise is an interdisciplinary challenge, requiring understanding of physiological chemistry and muscle physiology, and acid-base regulation. This Chapter will provide an introduction to this topic.

AEROBIC AND ANAEROBIC ASPECTS OF WORK PERFORMANCE

A. AEROBIC AND ANAEROBIC METABOLISM OF FUELS

The essence of the mechanism for movement of skeletal muscles is the temporary interaction between actin and myosin molecules. These are the key proteins in muscle cells for tension generation. The energy source closest to this interaction—regardless of whether lengthening, shortening, or static muscle tension occurs—is adenosine triphosphate (ATP). The free energy of hydrolysis of its terminal phosphate bond is sizable, and when the reaction shown below occurs in skeletal muscle cells:

$$\text{ATP} \rightarrow \text{ADP} + \text{inorganic phosphate} + \text{energy} \tag{1}$$

the energy released is available for the actin-myosin interactions.

Very little ATP actually exists in skeletal muscle, only about 6 mM/kg of wet weight—enough for perhaps one second of exercise energy. Thus, during exercise, ATP levels cannot decrease very much, because no surplus exists. Thanks to the presence of creatine phosphate (CP), a reservoir of phosphate existing in muscle, transphosphorylation allows ATP to be regenerated from ADP. This occurs as a result of the following equation, illustrating how phosphate bound to CP is transferred to ATP:

$$\text{ADP} + \text{CP} \xrightleftharpoons{\text{Creatine kinase}} \text{ATP} + \text{C} \tag{2}$$

Of course, CP must be regenerated using additional phosphate, obtained by more ATP production from metabolism of food.

Fatty acids and carbohydrates are equally efficient in providing energy for muscle tension generation if one considers the amount of free energy used as ATP bond energy. This is 1 ATP per 18.1 kCal (75.7 kJ) of free energy, be it from a carbohydrate such as glucose, or a fatty acid such as palmitic acid. However, even assuming that complete (aerobic) metabolism to CO_2 and H_2O occurs with both, as shown by the following equations for glucose ($C_6H_{12}O_6$) and palmitic acid ($C_{16}H_{32}O_2$):

$$C_6H_{12}O_6 + 6O_2 \rightarrow 6CO_2 + 6H_2O + 36 \text{ ATP} \tag{3}$$

$$C_{16}H_{32}O_2 + 23O_2 \rightarrow 16CO_2 + 16H_2O + 130\text{ATP} \tag{4}$$

fatty acids are about 10% less efficient in terms of energy provided per quantity of O_2 consumed.

The ratio between the amount of CO_2 produced in metabolism and the amount of O_2 used is called the *respiratory exchange ratio* (R). The R of carbohydrate is 1.00, that of fatty acids is close to 0.70. Since protein generally is not metabolized for energy during exercise, by monitoring R one can obtain an impression of the relative dominance of one or the other fuel source for energy. A typical resting R value is 0.80, indicating that free fatty acids are contributing the largest share of available energy.

Carbohydrates are the energy source in anaerobic metabolism; fatty acids are not metabolized anaerobically. No O_2 is utilized in anaerobic metabolism, and glucose is eventually converted to pyruvic acid. Excess pyruvic acid is stored temporarily as lactic acid *(Figure 12-1)*. This process yields very little energy— only 2 ATP per glucose instead of 38. Thus, 19 times more glucose must be metabolized anaerobically to produce an aerobic equivalent of ATP energy. Sprinters consume lavish quantities of energy anaerobically and accomplish their prodigious feats at the expense of developing metabolic acidosis, which very quickly brings debilitating fatigue. For endurance activity it is thus essential

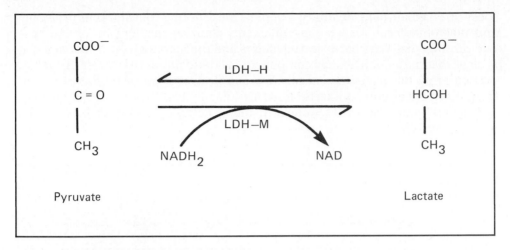

Figure 12-1. The enzyme lactic dehydrogenase (LDH) facilitates the intercon-
version of pyruvic and lactic acids, with reduced nicotinamide adenine dinucle-
otide ($NADH_2$) serving as the hydrogen donor when pyruvic acid is converted to
lactic acid. The LDH-H isoenzyme, found in heart and slow-twitch skeletal
muscle, preferentially favors the reaction proceeding toward pyruvic acid,
whereas the LDH-M form, present in fast-twitch skeletal muscles, favors the
reaction proceeding toward lactic acid.

that complete (aerobic) metabolism occur. This means the use of fatty acids as
well as a slower pace to permit adequate O_2 intake that minimizes accumulation
of metabolic acids.

Lactic acid in blood has a very low pK, and is more than 99% dissociated
into lactate$^-$ and H$^+$ ions. The bicarbonate system handles buffering of lactate
ions, as shown by the following equation:

$$\text{Lactate}^- + \text{H}^+ + \text{Na}^+ + \text{HCO}_3^- \rightleftarrows \text{Na-lactate} + \text{H}_2\text{CO}_3^- \rightleftarrows \text{H}_2\text{O} + \text{CO}_2 \tag{5}$$

Because CO_2, the acidic aspect of the buffer, is volatile, its loss via breathing
makes this buffer system very effective. Thus, the lungs and blood buffers are
effective at minimizing metabolic acid accumulation in the tissues. The elimination of lactic acid as CO_2 can be detected as an increase in the R (more CO_2
produced in relation to O_2 utilized). If blood HCO_3^- is measured at this same
time, it will have decreased. These changes represent the respiratory compensation to the metabolic acidosis of exercise.

The current interest in vigorous endurance-type exercise has brought with it
an increased awareness of the dynamics of energy metabolism when sizable
quantities of the body's fuel reserves are challenged. Scientists often use running
as an exercise modality to study endurance work, because there is minimum
contamination of performance variables by effects of equipment (as in cycling or
skiing), or special environments (as in swimming), or team sport skills (as in

soccer, basketball, etc.). Figure 12-2 depicts the differing contributions of aerobic and anaerobic metabolism to the total energy requirements for various competitive running distances between 100 meters and the marathon (42,195 meters). It is clear that the aerobic energy component is dominant for the longer distances, particularly 5,000 meters and greater. The simplest explanation for this resides in the performance-limiting effects of intracellular acidosis, which would increase significantly if inadequate O_2 were available for complete fuel metabolism in the working muscles.

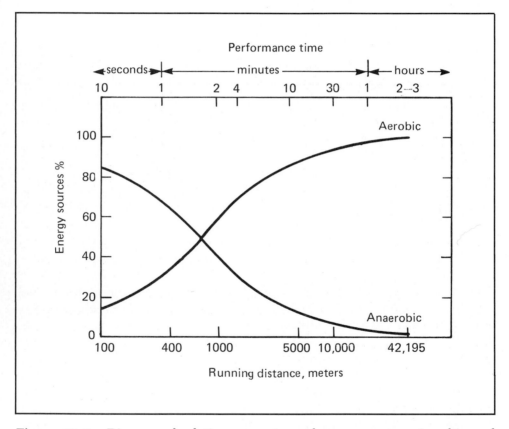

Figure 12-2.   Diagram of relative percentage of energy sources (aerobic and anaerobic) used covering various distances from sprinting to marathon running. As the running time increases, the need for adequate oxygen increases, otherwise the deleterious influence of metabolic acidosis will inhibit performance. (Reprinted with permission from Martin, D.E., G-O Dept. Bull., EUSM, 6(1):8, 1984.)

Any of the three primary foodstuffs—carbohydrates, fat, and protein—can be catabolized to yield ATP. Generally, fat and carbohydrate are considered as the usual sources except during starvation, when protein assumes an important role. During aerobic running, one will consume approximately 1 kcal/kg body weight/

km of distance. Thus, a marathon run for a 60 kg runner would have an energy requirement given by the following equation:

$$42.195 \text{ km} \times 1 \text{ kcal/kg/km} \times 60 \text{ kg} = 2,532 \text{ kcal (10,587 kJ)} \qquad (6)$$

If the runner were moving at a velocity of 7 min/mile (229 m/min), and thus able to finish the marathon in 3 hr 2 min, the energy consumption would be approximately 14 kcal/min (58.5 kJ/min). An elite athlete would consume approximately 20 kcal/min (83.6 kJ/min) and finish the race in about 2 hours and 11 minutes at a velocity of about 5 min/mile (322 m/min).

B. INCREASING WORK INTENSITY

As one increases the work rate, three major questions can be asked to determine whether aerobic metabolism can satisfy the energy requirements. First, do the muscle cells have enough mitochondrial enzymes to ensure complete breakdown of fuels? Second, since enzyme function is closely regulated by intracellular pH, will intermediate organic acid metabolites such as lactic acid limit the overall metabolic rate? Third, since the cytochrome enzyme system requires molecular O_2 to complete fuel catabolism and enormous energy release, will working muscle cells have adequate O_2? The answers to these questions depend, of course, on the intensity of exercise and extent of prior training. It appears that vigorous endurance training increases skeletal muscle cellular capabilities. There are more mitochondria, more mitochondrial and cytoplasmic enzymes for aerobic fuel breakdown, and more stored fuels. Better perfusion from an increased blood volume improves O_2 delivery and CO_2 removal, delaying the onset of acidosis in working muscles. The greater the duration or intensity of exercise, however, the more challenged these adaptations will be in their effectiveness.

At the organ system level, maintenance of an adequate O_2 supply going to the skeletal muscles requires the teamwork of three major mechanisms. First, lungs must ensure sufficient O_2 diffusion into the circulating blood. Second cardiac output must ensure adequate perfusion of tissues. Finally, there must be a rearrangement of blood flow, a preferential shunting to the working muscles.

Typically, the ability to perform endurance work, as indicated by one's maximum oxygen consumption rate ($\dot{V}O_2$-max) is measured using either a treadmill (Figure 12-3) or a bicycle ergometer test. The subject initially begins the test at a low, comfortable submaximal work rate; this is increased incrementally until either some predetermined target work rate is reached (a submaximal $\dot{V}O_2$ test) or the maximum achievable work rate occurs (a $\dot{V}O_2$-max test).

If one measures ventilation as ventilatory minute volume in ml/min ($\dot{V}_E$), one will observe a steadily increasing $\dot{V}_E$ as the workload increases. This is graphically depicted in Figure 12-4. Not only will the volume of O_2 consumed ($\dot{V}O_2$) increase, but also the volume of CO_2 produced ($\dot{V}CO_2$) will rise. During such an exercise stress test, typically lasting no more than 10 to 15 minutes, primarily glycogen from muscle is mobilized for energy rather than liver glycogen or blood glucose. As the exercise intensity increases, the R rises from its normal range of

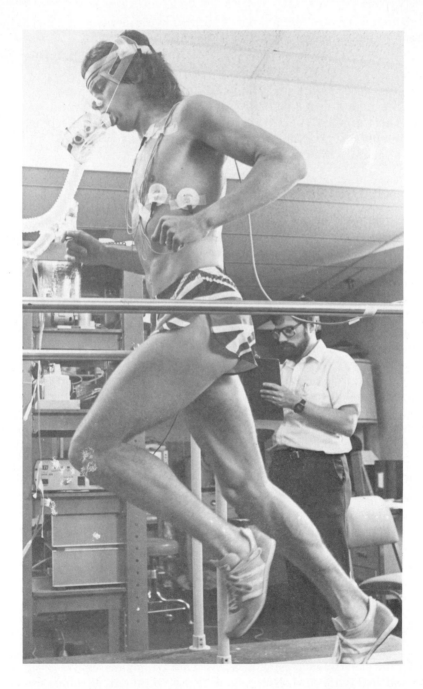

Figure 12-3. A treadmill stress test measures the oxygen uptake and carbon dioxide production, as well as other performance variables, during incrementally increasing work loads. Both submaximum and maximum intensities can be studied accurately. (Photograph courtesy of John Disney).

0.75 − 0.80, indicating the gradually greater emphasis on carbohydrate usage. There is a greater CO_2 production relative to O_2 utilized for carbohydrate as compared to fatty acid breakdown. As maximum oxygen uptake capabilities are achieved and surpassed, anaerobic metabolism will provide the added energy requirement. Accumulating H^+ ions from this metabolism will form additional CO_2 by shifting Equation (5) above preferentially to the right. This results not only in a reduction of blood bicarbonate buffer, but also increases the expired CO_2 levels more than can be explained by carbohydrate metabolism. R values will exceed 1.00 and such values are used as an indication that $\dot{V}O_2$-max has been achieved. Another criterion for $\dot{V}O_2$-max is an absence of increased O_2-uptake despite an increased work load.

THE RELATIONSHIP BETWEEN EXERCISE INTENSITY AND BLOOD LACTIC ACID LEVELS

A. THE CONCEPT OF ANAEROBIC THRESHOLD

The interrelationships between inadequate O_2 for metabolism and the production of metabolic acids (such as lactic) have been studied during most of the 20th century, and slowly the picture has unfolded. As long ago as 1907 Fletcher and Hopkins, using the frog gastrocnemius muscle, suggested that hypoxia induced lactic acid production when metabolism continued intensely. In the 1920s the British physiologist, A. V. Hill, came to the same conclusion. When he observed increased breathing following exercise, he coined the phase "O_2 debt" to imply this paying back of O_2 that was not available in sufficient quantities during exercise to prevent complete metabolism. Thus, it became customary to attempt quantitation of lactic acid production as a measure of anaerobiosis.

During the 1930s two groups, led by Margaria and Bang, using exercising men instead of frogs, observed an elevated blood lactic acid simultaneously with development of an O_2 debt during initial stages of an exercise bout. This clarified the cause-and-effect relationship between the two. Quantitation to estimate the intensity of exercise during the initial stages and during extended exercise indicated that a $\dot{V}O_2$ of about 1,800 to 2,500 ml/min would induce some anaerobic metabolism.

The factor explaining this metabolic acidosis centered primarily around cardiovascular limitations. Insufficient perfusion brought about inadequate muscle tissue oxygenation. In fact, this is not the complete story. Excessive glycogenolysis and glycolysis, involving breakdown of glycogen to glucose and finally to pyruvic acid, results in reduction of accumulating pyruvic acid to lactic acid. Thus, another factor involves the ability for these partially metabolized fuels to enter muscle cell mitochondria for complete oxidation.

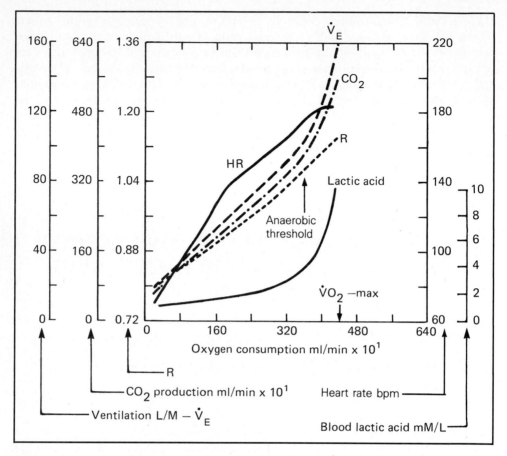

Figure 12-4. Graphic plot of increases in heart rate, $\dot{V}CO_2$, blood lactic acid and $\dot{V}_E$ observed in a distance runner during a treadmill stress test to determine maximum oxygen uptake. These variables are plotted as a function of increasing workload (here, increasing rate of oxygen consumption). Gradual shift in fuel-supply emphasis from free fatty acids to carbohydrates increases the R toward 1.0, with acidosis-induced $\dot{V}_E$ increases bringing it as high as 1.14. Minute ventilation ($\dot{V}_E$) reached nearly 160 liters per minute. Maximum heart rate peaked at 196 beats per minute. Maximum oxygen consumption was 4350 ml/min (with body weight of 58 kg, this was 75 ml/kg/min). At a $\dot{V}O_2$ of 3600 ml/min (also with blood lactic levels in the vicinity of 4 mM/L) the anaerobic threshold occurred (this is at 83% of $\dot{V}O_2$-max). These high-performance characteristics are typical of trained distance runners.

During the 1930s as well, parallel studies involving heart patients arrived at similar conclusions to those workers studying exercising muscle. Patients with acute heart failure had lowered arterial blood pH, which suggested that a hypoxic heart went into anaerobiosis, releasing lactic acid into the blood. Harrison and Pilcher studied the effects of exercise on patients with heart disease. They discovered higher R values in these patients during exercise than those observed in healthy people exercising at the same work load. They surmised that the hypoxic failing hearts were producing enough lactic acid that its diffusion into blood, with subsequent buffering by bicarbonate, increased the blood CO_2 concentration. The familiar bicarbonate buffering equation (5) was being shifted to the right as a result of increased blood H^+ ions from lactic acid metabolism.

Such investigations suggested that by any one of 2 measurements one could obtain an indication that anaerobic metabolism was occurring. The blood bicarbonate could be decreasing, and/or the expired volume of CO_2 ($\dot{V}CO_2$) could be increasing at a rate greater than that observed before this level of metabolism was achieved.

Thirty years later, in the 1960s, these concepts became the subject of renewed interest. Huckabee observed elevated blood lactic acid levels in patients with circulatory failure. Wasserman and McIlroy, in studies of exercising cardiac patients, found blood lactic acid levels rising out of proportion to blood pyruvic acid levels. Thus, the ratio of lactate to pyruvate ions increased. The obvious implication again was that the oxidative potential of the cardiac cells was decreased. A means was sought to better characterize this apparent anaerobic metabolic acidosis without resorting to frequent blood collections and lactic acid assays. They coined the term *anaerobic threshold* (AT) to describe the level of exercise $\dot{V}O_2$ above which aerobic energy production is supplemented by anaerobic mechanisms sufficiently that lactic acid levels begin to accumulate in arterial blood.

Early in the 1970s, Wasserman et al., suggested a non-invasive technique involving the monitoring of respiratory gas parameters, with computerized data analysis, as patients performed a gradually increasing intensity (incremental) work test on a bicycle ergometer. Ventilatory variables such as $\dot{V}O_2$, $\dot{V}CO_2$, $\dot{V}_E$, and R were plotted. When an abrupt but still linear departure from a previously linear increase in $\dot{V}CO_2$ or $\dot{V}_E$ occurred as the workload continued to increase, this was considered as the AT, corresponding to the threshold where lactic acid began to accumulate in the circulating blood. The ventilatory changes were simply a reflection of increased blood lactic acid levels. A somewhat similar graphic representation of data from a treadmill stress test of a distance runner, is shown in *Figure 12-4*.

This technique was modified for healthy subjects and athletes, using treadmills, by James Wilmore and David Costill, allowing study of not only AT but also $\dot{V}O_2$-max in individuals for whom running was more appropriate than cycling. This work was done during the early-to-mid 1970s, when a remarkable interest among Americans in improving physical fitness was stimulating considerable research in this aspect of sports medicine and exercise science. Costill and co-workers were among most active in this era to examine the physiological characteristics of trained distance runners, now possible by implementation of rapid-response gas analyzers and on-line computer analysis with graphic data presentation.

This technique of determining AT, $\dot{V}O_2$-max, and other physiological variables has been used extensively during the 1970s and 1980s in both exercise science and in cardiac rehabilitation medicine to evaluate physical fitness of a broad population, ranging from active athletes to sedentary people to patients with cardiac disease. Some workers have emphasized the use of gas exchange variables, while others have relied on blood collections to quantitate lactic acid levels. Many use both. Recent work has emphasized the careful analysis of results and ideas with a view toward learning more about the physiologic significance of AT and how it can be used in health and disease to monitor fitness.

B. PHYSIOLOGICAL SIGNIFICANCE OF THE ANAEROBIC THRESHOLD

Consideration of the meaning of the phrase "threshold of anaerobiosis" could in fact refer to two different concepts. Are we referring to an intracellular phenomenon whereby anaerobic metabolism begins to occur because of inadequate O_2 supplies? Or are we referring to a blood phenomenon whereby lactic acid levels therein begin to rise abruptly as a result of an ongoing accumulation?

The concept of AT does not imply a given work rate beyond which production of lactic acid in muscle or blood begins. Low intensities of exercise induce its production simply because never are all muscle cells in proximity to optimum blood perfusion, and some anaerobiosis occurs. Some lactic acid from these muscle cells diffuses out into the blood plasma, but it is removed as quickly as it is produced by both the active muscles themselves and by inactive muscle. The heart metabolizes sizable quantities of lactic acid during exercise. So does the liver and the kidney cortex. The muscles of trained athletes appear to convert pyruvic acid into alanine as well as to lactic acid. Thus, at relatively low work ratios, lactic acid is produced, and metabolized, but it doesn't accumulate.

It is, thus, appropriate to consider the AT as a work rate where blood lactic acid accumulation exceeds removal when compared to a previously equilibrated state. There is indeed the onset of a metabolic acidosis, but it is more indicative of a developing imbalance between the *equilibrium* of lactic acid production and metabolism than it is of the *initiation* of lactic acid production. Thus, acidification of the working skeletal muscles is occurring and lactic acid empties into the blood. This acid cannot be metabolized in comparable quantity by other tissues, and it starts to accumulate in the blood. The effects on pH of the dissociated H^+ ions from this lactic acid are minimal at the more moderate submaximum work loads because of excellent blood buffering mechanisms. When these are saturated, the accumulating H^+ ions then begin to decrease blood pH but also initiate an increase in ventilation. As seen in *Figure 11-4*, the work intensity at which an abrupt rise in blood lactic acid occurs is also one where $\dot{V}_E$ begins to increase at a faster rate than previously.

From a work performance viewpoint, AT is that intensity of work just below which effort can continue for extended periods without the onset of rapidly accumulating lactic acid concentration in the blood. Beyond the AT, the debilitating effects of increasing metabolic acidosis make long-term efforts at such intensity very difficult, eventually impossible. The activity threshold for rapid lactic acid accumulation in blood varies as a result of both training and genetic endowment. It may occur at work loads as low as 40% of $\dot{V}O_2$-max in untrained people, but at work loads as high as 80% to 90% of $\dot{V}O_2$-max in trained endurance athletes. Marathon runners typically race at their AT pace.

C. GENETIC VERSUS TRAINING EFFECTS IN ANAEROBIC THESHOLD DETERMINATION

Elite endurance athletes are genetically gifted for their excellence in performance. Effective adaptation to arduous training programs adds to this excellence. Knowledge of the difference between genetic and training factors provides a basis for understanding how the concepts of $\dot{V}O_2$-max and AT are affected by both.

A finding of essential importance in examining trained endurance athletes is that they have a greater absolute, as well as relative, reliance on oxidative phosphorylation (i.e., complete aerobic metabolism) even at high performance levels. Thus, by genetics or by training, they are aerobic specialists. Their muscle mitochondria have an increased oxidative enzyme capacity. Their muscle cells have an increased capillary density, ensuring better O_2 diffusion into cells. Their $\dot{V}O_2$-max is high, caused in part by a high maximal cardiac output and peripheral blood flow. Work by Andersen and Henriksson in particular has illustrated this increased aerobic potential. Following an 8 week training program, subjects having an average $\dot{V}O_2$-max increase of 16% also had comparable increases in capillary density (20%), but larger increases in succinic dehydrogenase and cytochrome oxidase activities (40%). Both of these mitochondrial enzymes are indicative of increased oxidative capabilities. Thus from an AT point of view, endurance-trained people, when compared to sedentary people, should be able to minimize blood lactic acid accumulation until relatively higher work rates are encountered. Endurance training thus can raise both $\dot{V}O_2$-max and AT.

An individual's skeletal muscle fiber type is of great importance in relation to lactic acid dynamics, because the various fiber types have different metabolic capabilities. Fiber type is genetically determined. Slow-twitch (ST) fibers, for example, have a lactic dehydrogenase (LDH) isoenzyme similar to that found in heart muscle (LDH-H), which predisposes toward pyruvate formation rather than lactate formation by keeping the reaction illustrated in *Figure 12-1* shifted toward the left. Slow-twitch fibers are sometimes called oxidative fibers because of their specialized abilities to permit complete fuel metabolism (more mitochondria, more myoglobin, better perfusion, etc.) Fast-twitch fibers (FT) are more specialized for glycolysis (anaerobic metabolism), and have an LDH iso-enzyme (LDH-M) which favors the reaction shown in *Figure 12-1* moving toward the right.

Some skeletal muscle fiber varieties have both oxidative (aerobic) and glycolytic capabilities well developed. These are termed FTb fibers to distinguish them from the other FT fibers, sometimes referred to as FTa, which preferentially are glycolytic in their metabolic preference. FTb fibers are less common, and possibly represent FTa fibers which have adapted to long-term endurance training by taking on ST (oxidative) properties. Apparently, ST fibers do not adapt similarly to strength training and take on FT properties.

It is not surprising that well-trained endurance athletes are genetically endowed with a preponderance of ST fibers. These fibers, because of their increased mitochondrial density and volume, are more specialized for breakdown of fatty acids. When such fuels are oxidized at a high rate, glycolysis is correspondingly slowed and lactic acid formation is diminished. Trained endurance athletes thus do not accumulate lactic acid in their blood until relatively high work rates in comparison to non-athletic sedentary people. This is due not only to the genetic component of skeletal muscle fiber type, but as well to training effects that increase the oxidative potential of their skeletal muscle fibers.

Another aspect in addition to training and genetic affects on performance is that different fiber types are recruited into action depending upon work intensity. Thus, ST fibers are typically recruited at lower work rates, FT fibers as well at higher rates.

D. PERCEIVED EXERTION AND BLOOD ACIDITY

One of the important end results of the glycogen-conserving aspect of endurance fitness (i.e., preferential use of free fatty acids) is that more work can be performed prior to carbohydrate stores being exhausted. This is significant because our perception of fatigue seems to correlate more with blood glucose levels than with fatty acid levels.

No one understands exactly the mechanism by which we perceive the intensity of hard work. Using the scale of rated perceived exertion (RPE) devised by Gunnar Borg, which rates exercise stress on a numerical scale of 1 to 18 as well as on a scale of descriptors, young adults perceive exercise at their AT as "somewhat hard" or 12. Burke's work indicates that a work load having a RPE level of 12 to 15 ("somewhat hard" to "hard") is useful for exercise prescription. At this intensity people are working at between 60% and 85% of their $\dot{V}O_2$-max and between 70% and 90% of their maximum heart rate. Other studies have indicated that improvements in endurance activity can occur by training in this range. The AT ranges from about 50% of $\dot{V}O_2$-max in untrained people to greater than 80% of $\dot{V}O_2$ max in elite athletes. Thus, there may be some prescriptive value in having people use RPE estimates of performance at AT as a basis for training.

The explanation for RPE of endurance work is most likely multifaceted. Blood lactic acid levels relate to sensation of effort when elevated. But so does ventilatory effort, with hyperventilation in vigorous exercise eventually resulting in the sensation of dyspnea when of sufficient magnitude. Thus, both local cues from the metabolic acidosis in muscle, and central cues from the cardiorespiratory system, interact.

ADAPTATIONS OF THE PULMONARY SYSTEM TO ENDURANCE EXERCISE

A. STRENGTH VERSUS ENDURANCE TRAINING OF VENTILATORY MUSCLES

An interesting question is whether the muscles of ventilation can improve their strength or endurance as a result of specific training. Improved ventilatory muscle endurance would imply that higher intensities of breathing could be sustained for a longer period. More ventilatory muscle strength would permit greater pressures when static, maximum-effort inspiratory and expiratory efforts are attempted. Since other skeletal muscles adapt positively to specific training, one could surmise that the ventilatory muscles respond similarly. As an example, does an endurance runner's normal ventilatory stimulus increase ventilatory system function, or is this training capable of being handled by existing ventilating abilities without further adaptive improvements? Would specific ventilatory muscle training bring improved abilities to perform?

Studies in my laboratory have evaluated trained endurance runners to determine whether their arduous training programs, which involve weekly running distances as high as 80 to 100 miles for months on end, secondarily improve ventilatory performance. A complicating factor in evaluating the pulmonary function variables of such athletes is that, without similar data from these same subjects acquired prior to their beginning such rigorous training, the influence of any contributing genetic components are unidentifiable. At present, other studies provide no evidence suggesting this to be an important source of error.

Among such trained male endurance runners, there appear to be notable increases (when compared to sedentary people) in MVV, in peak expiratory flow rate (PEFR), and in pulmonary diffusing capacity (D_LCO) as measured using a single-breath test. Changes in MVV and PEFR could be explained simply by elevated aerobic capabilities of the major muscles used in breathing, particularly the diaphragm and abdominal muscles. Calisthenic exercises such as repeat bouts of situps to increase abdominal muscle performance are a typical accompaniment to the daily training assignment of running for a specific distance and at a given intensity.

The increase in resting D_LCO is perhaps also explainable. There are two aspects to consider. One concerns the membrane component of this variable, determined by the thickness, physicochemical properties, and surface area of the alveolocapillary membrane. We do not know that these aspects change with endurance training. In runners, lung volumes do not appear to increase. The other aspect relates to the perfusion component of D_LCO. Remember that D_LCO indicates the ease of exchange of alveolar gases across the alveolocapillary membrane, through the blood plasma, and into the erythrocytes with their hemoglobin molecules. Although the evidence is not in uniform agreement, it appears likely that endurance training brings about an increase in blood volume (both plasma and erythrocytes), which in turn should increase the resting pulmonary blood volume, thus providing more functional diffusional area for alveolar gas exchange with blood. Mild endurance training is minimal in eliciting such adaptive changes, however, since the challenge provided to the ventilatory system by jogging is quite easily met by the existing performance capabilities of the chest-lung system. An adaptive reserve, however, can apparently become functional when developed through arduous training.

B. SPECIFIC TRAINING OF VENTILATORY MUSCLES

One major problem in studying this topic is that a great many different muscle groups contribute to ventilation at increased workloads. Each of these muscle groups has its own physiologic properties, notably determined by the relative percentage of fast-twitch and slow-twitch fibers. The diaphragm always plays a very important role in inspiration, however, and it has been well-studied. Typically in humans it is comprised of roughly 55% slow-twitch, 20% fast-twitch type a (emphasis on glycolytic metabolism), and 25% fast-twitch type b (fast in tension generation but with both oxidative and glycolytic capabilities). Thus, this muscle has both strength-oriented and endurance-oriented characteristics from its generous endowment with, respectively, fast-twitch and slow-twitch fibers. Indeed, studies by David Leith and Mark Bradley have suggested that specific strength or endurance training of ventilatory muscles will improve their performance as measured by appropriate pulmonary function test variables. It is presumed that the other accessory muscles of breathing, with their own unique mix of FT and ST fibers, adapt along with the diaphragm.

What kinds of pulmonary function test variables are changed with each type of training? Leith and Bradley found that specific strength training increased maximum inspiratory and expiratory pressures. Endurance training increased maximum voluntary ventilation (MVV) over 15 seconds as well as the maximum sustainable voluntary ventilation (MSVV) over 15 minutes. The subjects for their study, however, engaged over a 5-week period specifically in training maneuvers which challenged their ventilatory muscles. In a real sense, then, a specific training stimulus was applied.

In clinical medicine, such variables as MVV and PEFR can be increased in patients with chronic obstructive pulmonary disease. In a sense such patients are faced with a dilemma similar to that of a vigorously exercising athlete, i.e., an increased requirement to manage the chest-lung dynamics of increased ventilation. For a long distance runner, however, this requirement may continue for only a few hours; it is nonstop in patients with serious obstructive lung disease. The development of small, easy-to-use, inspiratory resistive breathing devices has allowed such patients to improve tolerance to routine breathing workloads, with reduced sensations of dyspnea. In some reports, specific improvements in clinically measured variables such as MVV are observed.

RELEVANT READING

Asmussen, E., and Nielsen, M. Studies on the regulation of respiration in heavy work. *Acta Physiologica Scandinavica* **12**:171–178, 1946.

Bang, O. The lactate content of the blood during and after muscular exercise in man. *Scand Arch Physiol* **74**(Suppl):49–82, 1936.

Borg, G.A.V. Perceived exertion: A note on history and methods. *Medicine and Science in Sports* **5**:90–93, 1973.

Bouhuys, A., Pool, J., Binkhurst, R.A., and Leeuwen, P.V. Metabolic acidosis of exercise in healthy males. *Journal of Applied Physiology* **21**:1040–1046, 1966.

Burke, E.F. Individualized fitness program using perceived exertion for the prescription of healthy adults. *Journal of Physical Education and Recreation* **49**:35–37, 1979.

Cain, D.V., Infante, A.A., and Davies, R.E. Chemistry of muscle contraction. Adenosine triphosphate and phosphocreatine as energy supplies for single contractions of working muscles. *Nature* **196**:214–217, 1962.

Costill, D.L., and Fox, E.L. Energetics of marathon running. *Medicine and Science in Sports* **1**:81–86, 1969.

Diamant, B., Karlson, J., and Saltin, B. Muscle tissue lactate after maximal exercise in man. *Acta Physiologica Scandinavica* **72**:383–384, 1968.

Farrell, P., Wilmore, J.M., Coyle, E.F., Billing, I.E., and Costill, D.L. Plasma lactate accumulation and distance running performance. *Medicine and Science ·in Sports and Exercise* **11**:338–344, 1979.

Harrison, T.R., and Pilcher, C. Studies in congestive heart failure. II. The respiratory exchange during and after exercise. *Journal of Clinical Investigation* **8**:291–315, 1930.

Holloszy, J. Adaptations of muscle tissue to training. *Progress in Cardiovascular Disease* **8**:445–458, 1976.

Huckabee, W.E. Abnormal resting blood lactate. I. The significance of hyperlactatemia in hospitalized patients. *American Journal of Medicine* **30**:833–839, 1961.

Ivy, J., Withers, R., Van Handel, P., Elger, D., and Costill, D. Muscle respiratory capacity and fiber type as determinants of the lactate threshold. *Journal of Applied Physiology* **48**:523–527, 1980.

Jones, N.L., and Ehrsam, R.E. The anaerobic threshold. *Exercise and Sports Sciences Reviews* **10**:49–83, 1982.

Jorfeldt, L., Dannfelt, A., and Karlsson, J. Lactate release in relation to tissue lactate in human skeletal muscle during exercise. *Journal of Applied Physiology* **44**:350–352, 1978.

Lafontaine, T.P., Londeree, B.R., and Spath, W.L. The maximal steady state versus selected running events. *Medicine and Science in Sports and Exercise* **13**:190–192, 1981.

Leith, D.E., and Bradley, M. Ventilatory muscle strength and endurance training. *Journal of Applied Physiology* **41**:508–516, 1976.

Mader, A., Liesen, H., Heck, H., Philippi, H., Rost, R., Schurch, P., and Hollmann, W. Zur Beurteilung der sportarztspecifischen Ausdauerleistungsfahigkeit im Labor. *Sportarzt and sportmedizin* **27**:80–88, 109–112, 1976.

Margaria, R., Edwards, H.T., and Dill, D.B. The possible mechanisms of contracting and paying the oxygen debt and role of lactic acid in muscular contraction. *American Journal of Physiology* **106**:689–715, 1933.

Martin, D.E. Performance of women in endurance sports: interaction of cardiopulmonary with other physiological parameters. *Gynecology-Obstetrics Dept. Bulletin, Emory Univ. School of Medicine* **6**(1):5–20, 1984.

Martin, D.E., Vroon, D.H., May, D.F., and Pilbeam, S.P. Physiological changes in elite male distance runners training for Olympic competition. *Physician and Sportsmedicine* **16**(1):152–171, 1986.

Martin, D.E., May, D.F., and Pilbeam, S.P. Ventilation limitations to performance among elite male distance runners. *The 1984 Olympic Scientific Congress Proceedings Vol. 3. Sport and Elite Performers*, (D.M. Landers, ed.), pp. 121–131, 1986.

Owles, W.H. Alterations in the lactic acid content of the blood as a result of light exercise and associated changes in the CO_2 combining power of the blood and in the alveolar CO_2 pressure. *Journal of Physiology* **69**:214–237, 1930.

Rowell, L.B., Kraning, K.K., Evans, T.O., Kennedy, J.W., Blackmon, J.R., and Kusami, F. Splanchnic removal of lactate and pyruvate during prolonged exercise in man. *Journal of Applied Physiology* **21**:1773–1783, 1966.

Skinner, J.S., and McLellan, T.H. The transition from aerobic to anaerobic metabolism. *Research Quarterly* **51**:234–248, 1980.

Sonne, L.J., and Davis, J.A. Increased exercise performance in patients with severe COPD following inspiratory resistive training. *Chest* **81**:436–439, 1982.

Thorstensson, A., Sjodin, B., Tesch, P., and Karlsson, J. Actomyosin ATP-ase, myokinase, CPK, and LDH in human fast and slow twitch muscle fibers. *Acta Physiologica Scandinavica* **99**:225–229, 1977.

Wasserman, K., and McIlroy, M.B. Detecting the threshold of anaerobic metabolism in cardiac patients during exercise. *American Journal of Cardiology* **14**:844–852, 1964.

Wasserman, K., Whipp, B.J., Koyal, S.N., and Beaver, W.L. Anaerobic threshold and respiratory gas exchange during exercise. *Journal of Applied Physiology* **35**:236–243, 1973.

Wasserman, K. The anaerobic threshold measurement to evaluate exercise performance. *American Review of Respiratory Disease* **129**:(Suppl.)S35–S40, 1984.

Wilmore, J.H., and Costill, D. Semi-automated systems approach to the assessment of oxygen uptake during exercise. *Journal of Applied Physiology* **36**:618–620, 1974.

Withers, R.T., Sherman, W.M. Miller, J.M., and Costill, D.L. Specificity of the anaerobic threshold in endurance trained cyclists and runners. *European Journal of Applied Physiology* **47**:93–104, 1981.

INDEX